CREATING HEALTH

WITH REAL FOOD

Proven Strategies to Slow Aging,
Control Weight, and Prevent or
Reverse Most Diseases

Andrea Covert, Ph.D.

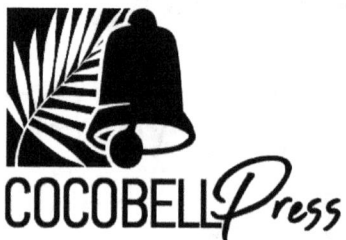

CREATING HEALTH

WITH REAL FOOD

Proven Strategies to Slow Aging,
Control Weight, and Prevent or
Reverse Most Diseases

Andrea Covert, Ph.D.

COCOBELL*Press*

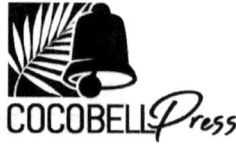

This book is based on research and the opinions of the author. The author of this book is not giving medical or other professional advice to the individual reader. This book is not meant to prescribe the use of any technique as a form of diagnosis or treatment for any physical, emotional or medical condition. The intent of the author is to offer information to help the reader make informed decisions about his or her health. This information is not meant as a substitute for the advice of your doctor. If the reader chooses to use the information in this book, the author and publisher assume no responsibility for the consequences. The author disclaims any liability with respect to any loss, injury, or damage arising directly or indirectly from the use of this book. The reader should consult his or her licensed health care practitioner before using any suggestions in this book.

Mention of any companies or people is not meant as an endorsement by the author or publisher.

Names: Andrea Covert, Ph.D., author.
Title: Creating Health with Real Food: Proven Strategies to Slow Aging, Control Weight, and Prevent or Reverse Most Diseases
First Published by Cocobell Press in 2021
3298 Governor Dr., San Diego, CA. 92192.

Printed in the United States of America.
ISBN 978-1-7374207-0-5 (print), ISBN 978-1-7374207-1-2 (ebook).
First Edition
Revised and updated February, 2024
Cover design: Vincent Saldana
Proofreaders: Robert Labelle, James Taylor, Sally Tang, and Keziah Daniel

Dedicated to my sweetheart, Robert, who has patiently listened to me talk about my journey towards lifelong health and longevity. Without your steady love and support, I could not have written this book.

And to all of my grandchildren. My hope is you take an interest in lifelong health: Alison, Annabelle, Carter, Colette, Corbin, Chloe, Kyle, Luke, Mackenzie, Rex, Ryatt, and Sophie. I thought of you often as I wrote this book.

Contents

Introduction

These are the questions I wanted to find the answers to

Weight:

- What causes weight gain?
- How can I lose weight without being constantly hungry?
- How can I control weight gain?

Health and long life:

- What do I need to eat to live a long and healthy life?
- How can I avoid a heart attack and stroke?
- How can I avoid brain deterioration, such as Alzheimer's?

Disease:

- What causes diseases?
- How can I heal myself if I get sick?

What else besides food matters for a long healthy life?

- Exercise
- Sleep
- Stress
- Mental health
- Relationships
- A purpose in life

I succeeded in answering all of these questions. My journey through the research and my personal journey are documented in this book. I hope this information will be as transformative for you as it has been for me.

Why I wrote this book

I spent six years reviewing research to figure out what science has to say about how to have excellent health right up to the end of life.

I wanted to know what to eat that would lead to:

- **No strokes**
- **No cardiovascular disease**
- **No cancer**
- **No disease**
- **A sharp brain**
- **A body that still works well**
- **No pain**
- **No need for medication**
- **Easy control over my weight and hunger**

I did figure out how to do all of these things. The answer, according to research, is not what you have been told by the government and probably not by your doctor.

I have a Ph.D. I understand research. I understand how to read research to determine if the results are meaningful.

What were the results of this research? A diet that was very much like the popular "keto" diet.

That is a high-fat, low-carbohydrate diet combined with intermittent fasting (eating one big meal per day, and leaving more time between meals).

What did I change? I added more healthy fats (eliminating vegetable and seed oils), eliminated sugar and most sweeteners, and eliminated grains. I always ate a lot of vegetables, and still do. I eat less fruit now, because of the sugar content.

My hunger is completely manageable now that I eat more fat and have reduced my carbs. In addition, I have lost my cravings for sweets and other carbohydrates, and it is easy to maintain my weight.

I am 75, have no pain, take no medication, and still lead a

very active lifestyle.

I should point out that:

- No one paid me to write this book.
- I sell no products.
- I have no reason to bias the results I have come up with.
- I wrote this book as a gift to anyone who wants to be healthy.

Chapter 1

Overview

We are an amazing species

We can live almost anywhere and thrive. The Eskimos live in the ice and snow in Alaska. The Australian aborigines live in scorching heat in the desert.

We can eat almost anything. There are people who eat only animal products, like the Eskimos who eat things like fish and seals, and virtually no vegetables. There are the Maasai in Africa where the male warriors consume only milk, meat, and blood from their cattle. Then there is the village up in the hills of Okinawa where they eat 98% plants, including 67% sweet potatoes. [1]

We are amazingly adaptable.

Our bodies want to be healthy, and they have an impressive array of mechanisms to keep us that way. For example, if we eat salt, our bodies hold more water to keep our salt balance within a very narrow range.

However, there are limits to the adaptability of our bodies.

Our bodies need certain basic things to do well.

What do our bodies need to thrive?

- **Clean air**
- **Healthy water**
- **Food with adequate nutrition**
- **No added poison to any of these**
- **Sunshine**
- **Move 30-45 minutes per day**
- **Healthy relationships**
- **Purpose in life**

Generally, we had all of these available in abundance just a few hundred years ago. Now, not so much.

If you could magically have all of these things, even for just a month, this is what you might expect:

- Probably lose weight.
- Have more energy.
- Sleep better.
- Be happier.

What's possible from healthy living?

If you continue with this program, as you go through life, you will probably experience most, if not all, of the following:

Physically:

- Easier to maintain a **healthy weight**.
- Have **strong muscles** to do your favorite activities.
- Have a **stronger immune system** (very few illnesses, such as colds and flu).
- Have **more energy**, so you will feel like doing things.
- Have very **few aches and pains**
- **Age more slowly.**
- Have a healthier **digestive system**.
- **Sleep better.**
- Have no or **limited acne** as a teen.
- Have healthier **skin color** throughout life.
- Develop fewer **wrinkles** as you age.

- Have **hair that stays thicker and healthier** longer, and maintains its **color longer** before turning grey.
- **Live longer** and remain disease-free right up until you die.
- **Not develop "diseases of affluence"**, or if you have them, they might be reversed or at least slowed down. Diseases of affluence are diseases that appear as cultures become more affluent and begin abandoning their indigenous diets, and instead begin to eat processed and packaged foods.

Some examples of these "diseases of affluence" are:

Heart disease	Digestive disorders
Cancer	Depression
Alzheimer's	Mood disorders
Obesity	Brain fog
Multiple Sclerosis (MS)	Sleep disorders
Autoimmune diseases	Autism
Arthritis	Diabetes

Mentally:

- **Be more alert.**
- Be **less depressed.**
- Be **more joyful.**
- Have a **better memory.**
- **Be less sleepy during the day.**
- **Avoid "brain fog".**
- **Your brain will work well right up until you die.**

I am not guaranteeing that everyone will get these results. There are genetic differences that can influence our health. **It is estimated that 10-50% of health is genetic** (depending on the gene). That leaves 50-90% that is under our control. (See section on genes.)

Are we taking good care of our bodies now?

- Our public drinking water has added chlorine, and 70% of our water has glyphosate (the poison that is the main ingredient in Roundup).

- Our food generally has very little nutrition compared to 100 years ago, due to factory farming and eating processed foods.
- We cover ourselves when we go outside with hats and sunscreen, so we get very little sunshine on our skin (important for Vitamin D).
- Our relationships are deteriorating. We live isolated lives. When we go out, many of us are on our cell phones rather than talking to each other. The quality of our relationships has an impact on our general health.

In addition, we are adding poison to our environment:

- Our air is polluted.
- We are destroying ocean habitats. Our oceans are so polluted with mercury that most fish are too unhealthy for us to eat.
- We have added 1.8 million tons of glyphosate (the primary poison in Roundup) to our food here in America, and 9.4 million tons worldwide since its introduction in 1974 [2].

What has that done to our health? An explosion of chronic diseases.

The good news is that we have the power to prevent and/or reverse these diseases. If we take excellent care of our bodies, the gene for any particular disease may never show up. If we abuse our bodies, genes may determine which disease we get. In other words, whatever your genetic weak spot is, that disease will show up first.

Perhaps we can prevent or reverse diseases if we take control of our health. If too much damage has already been done, the disease may not be completely reversible, but you don't know until you try.

If we take excellent care of our bodies, we should be able to be healthy right up to the day we die, at a very old age. Our brains should work, our bodies should be disease-free, and we should have abundant energy to do the fun things we want to do.

How long can we live if we take good care of ourselves? Many people who do this live into their nineties, and sometimes even over 100, in good health.

Jack LaLanne is a good example of this. He was a sickly child. This is how he described it: "As a kid, I was a sugarholic and a junk food junkie! It made me weak and it made me mean. It made me so sick I had boils, pimples and suffered from nearsightedness. Little girls used to beat me up."[12]

He decided to change his ways. He started exercising two hours every day. He changed how he ate. His motto: "If man made it, don't eat it." [12]

He lived until 96. According to his family, he had been sick only for about a week, but continued to do his daily workout routine right up to the day before he died.

He died of pneumonia. Not cancer, not a heart attack and not one of the other diseases that are a result of poor lifestyle choices.

What we are currently doing is not working

"Leave your drugs in the chemist's pot
if you can cure the patient with food."
--Hippocrates

Americans are getting sicker and sicker. The obesity rate is now 38%. Fifty per cent of Americans are diabetic or pre-diabetic. Heart disease and cancer are now the leading causes of death.

In 1900, heart disease and cancer accounted for only 12% of all deaths. By 2010, that skyrocketed to 47% of all deaths.

Processed food looks and tastes like food, but it really isn't. It is calories, but not only does it have very little nutrition, but it is toxic. It literally contains poison (primarily glyphosate, the main ingredient in Roundup). It is slowly killing us.

Many of the diseases that we have today are largely preventable or even reversible through food and lifestyle changes.

Eliminating sugar, flour, seed and bean oils, and the processed foods made from these foods is a good start.

What does work?

What most research agrees on:

- Do not eat processed or packaged food. A very few are OK. Check the labels.
- Eat only organic "real food".

- Do not eat deep-fried food.
- Do not eat heavily processed vegetable oils (corn oil, cottonseed oil, soybean oil, safflower oil, rapeseed oil, canola oil, or foods that contain them).
- Eat a good variety of organic fruits, vegetables, nuts and seeds every day -- mostly vegetables.

Pretty easy rules.

What research does not agree on:

- Whether to eat meat, dairy or other animal products.
- How much fat to eat. It ranges from 0- 60% or more of calories. Wow! That's quite a range.
- How much saturated fat to eat. The range is from zero to unlimited.
- How much starchy carbohydrates, such as beans, grains, bread, pasta, and potatoes, to eat. The range is from zero to a moderate amount.

Some of the most popular diets

My comments are in italics.

- **Vegan diet.** Just fruit, vegetables, and grains. No animal products such as dairy, fish, or meat. *Adequate protein may be a problem. Remember to take B12 and K2 supplements.*
- **Vegetarian diet.** Fruits, vegetables, and grains, but no meat or fish. Some animal products such as dairy and eggs are acceptable. *This may work for many people.*
- **Pescatarian.** The same as a vegetarian, but eating fish is acceptable. *Because of the healthy omega-3 fats and healthy protein, this is probably a great diet to keep people healthy.*
- **Paleo diet.** Meat, fat, and vegetables. No dairy, grains, or beans. Only eat food that may have existed in primitive times (or at least our modern equivalent). Loren Cordain writes about this diet. *Similar to a high fat, low carb diet, but it may contain more meat. Excess protein can become glucose (bad) -- see chapter on protein.*

- **Carnivore diet.** No vegetables, fruit, grains, or dairy. Just meat and animal fat, preferably eating the animal "nose to tail", including the liver. Some people do well on this, especially if they have many food allergies. Some people who cannot lose weight any other way are successful on this diet. Dr. Paul Saladino is a good source of information for this diet. *This may work well, but I am concerned about the micronutrients in vegetables and fruits. I think it is safer to eat a range of fruits and vegetables, in part to keep our microbiome healthy (more on this later).*
- **Low fat, high carb (LFHC)** The most extreme supporter of this group is Caldwell Esselstein (see section on reversing diseases). He suggests eliminating all fats, even avocadoes, nuts, and seeds. Starchy vegetables and grains are fine.
- **High fat, low carb (HFLC)** This diet encourages people to eat a high percentage of calories from healthy fats, including saturated animal fats. Most of the food should be non-starchy vegetables, with very few, or no starchy vegetables (such as potatoes), sugars, or grains. Animal proteins and fish are acceptable. Atkins is the most famous proponent of this diet.

(Personal Note)

After reading research for several years, and trying all of these diets, which one worked the best for me? The high fat, low carbohydrate diet (HFLC).

We all have different bodies. Try different ways of eating and see what works for you. However, all experts seem to agree that we should be eliminating packaged and processed foods, and eating only real foods. No deep-fried foods. Limit or eliminate sugar, and processed vegetable oils.

Just doing that much will probably make a huge difference in your health.

Let's look at high fat, low carbohydrates (HFLC) more carefully.

Do eat:

- All meats, including beef, chicken, and pork (excluding processed meats).

- All parts of the animal, such as the liver, and the fat.
- Avocados (high in healthy fat).
- Nuts and seeds (high in healthy fat).
- Full-fat dairy, including full-fat milk (whole milk), cheese, sour cream, cream cheese, and yogurt.
- Unlimited amounts of non-starchy vegetables (at least 60% of food by volume).
- Limited amount of fruits (due to sugar content).
- Low-sugar fruits, such as blueberries.
- Healthy oils, such as olive oil, coconut oil, avocado oil, and healthy animal fats.

Do not eat:

- Seed or bean oils, such as canola oil, soybean oil, corn oil, safflower oil, rapeseed oil, and cottonseed oil.
- Grains such as wheat, barley, corn, and rye.
- Bread.
- Pasta.
- Pizza crust.
- Beans.
- Potatoes.
- Fruit with high sugar content, such as grapes.
- Large amounts of fruit, due to the high sugar content.
- Sugar in any form, even the more natural sugars, such as agave nectar, honey, and maple syrup.
- Artificial sweeteners.
- Processed or packaged foods.

What are processed and packaged foods? Do not eat these.

- Anything in a package or box (one ingredient is OK, such as whole milk)
- Anything with an ingredient list (unless it is just one food, such as cheese, which may have whole milk, salt and cheese culture or enzymes to make the cheese)
- All fast foods (some salad bars may be OK if they have fresh real food)
- Potato chips

- Corn chips
- Bread
- Cookies
- Candy
- Cakes
- Cupcakes
- Doughnuts
- Deep fried foods
- Breakfast cereals
- Muffins
- Bagels
- Pizza crust made with flour
- Oatmeal in a package, especially with added sugar
- Processed meats such as pepperoni, sausage, or cold cuts
- Canned fruits and vegetables
- Frozen dinners (frozen fruits and vegetables are fine if they have nothing added)
- Yogurt that has any added ingredients, such as fruit and sugar
- Chocolate milk (because of the added sugar)
- All sodas with real or artificial sugars
- Sports drinks
- All processed seed and bean oils, commonly called "vegetable oils". Olive oil, coconut oil and avocado are fine.
- Cheese that has added ingredients other than salt, enzymes and starter culture
- Almost everything in the grocery that is not in the fresh produce section
- Most sugars, including table sugar, brown sugar, maple syrup, agave nectar, and honey
- Sugars that are hidden in ingredients lists such as dextrose, maltose, sucrose, and lactose
- All artificial sweeteners
- Biscuits
- Crackers
- Pasta if made with wheat flour
- Rice
- Jellies, jams, and preserves
- Sauces and gravies thickened with flour or cornstarch
- Beer
- Sweet wines and liqueurs

- Table salt (natural salts, such as sea salts, are good for us)

Some few packaged foods are OK. Read the ingredient list. All ingredients should be real food.

Note that all diets, expect the carnivore diet, encourage unlimited amounts of non-starchy vegetables. These should be 60-80 percent of our food by volume, no matter what diet you follow. Non-starchy vegetables are low in calories, high in fiber, and high in nutrition.

Some common non-starchy vegetables

Onions, Broccoli, Carrots, Celery, Cucumber, Green beans, Cabbage, Fennel, Leeks, Mushrooms, Asparagus, Beets, Brussel sprouts, Cabbage, Collard greens, Bell pepper, Green peas, Kale, Spinach, Tomatoes,Watercress, Lettuce, Garlic, Ginger, Oregano, Cilantro, Parsley, Basil, Thyme, Rosemary, Sage, and All sprouts

---

Different diets work for different people. We have different genes, differences in microbiome, varied exposure to antibiotics or toxins.

The most important change you can make is to eat real food.

The Standard American Diet (SAD)

Most people in America are eating the Standard American Diet. What is this?

If you are eating:

- **Anything you want**
- **As much as you want**
- **Whenever you want**

Then you are eating the Standard American Diet. More on this later.

Not everyone who knows what to eat will want change. However, I have written this book for people who want to be healthy but just don't know how.

I also have videos online on how to cook. They are for excellent cooks, and for people who do not know how to cook at all. I show how to chop, cook, store and make incredibly delicious food.

My system is very simple. My recipes are all from ingredients that are readily available. In addition, I have listed exactly where I buy things.

I think my food is really delicious. I love food. I love delicious food. I actually prefer eating my healthy food.

If you get used to this food, I predict that you will no longer want most of the Standard American Diet (SAD). In fact, you will wonder why you ever ate it.

Combine this great food with exercise, and WOW!! You will be amazed at how great your body can feel.

You can go "cold turkey" and just change, or you can start little by little, one meal at a time. Do what works for you.

In this book I have included:

- A general review of the research literature on healthy eating
- What else to do to stay healthy
- Recipes

I recommend you watch *Forks Over Knives* and *Fat, Sick and Nearly Dead*. They reflect a vegan diet, which is not what I do, but it is still very interesting information. It is clear in these movies that most major illnesses are completely reversible. Other good movies are *The Magic Pill* and *Food as Medicine*, 2016.

Also, go on YouTube and search for Mark Hyman, Terry Wahls, Jason Fung, Sten Ekberg, or Joseph Mercola. Watch their videos. They are all very informative and entertaining. They base their recommendations on research. They do not have the same ideas about what to eat, but they agree on most things.

Dr. Mercola also has an excellent free daily email newsletter. *Dr. Mercola.com*

I list the experts in each field. Look these people up on YouTube and watch their lectures. Most lectures are presented to general audiences and are very watchable. If you want a more academic approach, look for lectures given to professional audiences. We are so lucky to get to listen to the experts in each field right there on the internet! The other option is to buy their books, or check them out of the library.

Take Away

- We are an amazing species that can eat almost anything and live almost anywhere.
- What we are currently doing is not working. We are destroying our health, and damaging our environment.
- We have the power to become healthy, primarily by changing what we eat.

Chapter 2

Maintaining Our Ideal Weight

Doing the research for this chapter allowed me to have total control over my weight for the first time in my life. The main thing I learned is that insulin is primarily what controls weight gain and loss, not calories, although calories do matter. Read on to find out how this works.

"In our body, nothing happens by accident. Every single physiological process is a tight orchestration of hormonal signals. Whether our heart beats faster or slower is tightly controlled by hormones. Whether we urinate a lot or a little is tightly controlled by hormones. Whether the calories we eat are burned as energy or stored as body fat is also tightly controlled by hormones. So, the main problem in terms of obesity is not the number of calories we eat, but how they are spent. And the main hormone we need to know about is insulin."

--Jason Fung [3]

One of our primary concerns is losing weight.

The top three New Year's resolutions in 2019 were:

1. Diet or eat healthier (71%)
2. Exercise more (65%)
3. Lose weight (54%) [4]

No one wants to be fat. And yet, many of us seem almost powerless to control our weight. Why is that?

Overview of the problem

What we are eating is a problem. The American diet consists of 63% processed food, primarily made up of sugar, flour, and unhealthy vegetable oils.

When we eat a diet high in carbohydrates (flour, sugar, and starchy vegetables, like potatoes), our blood sugar spikes, and then it crashes. The crash creates cravings for more carbohydrates. We end up craving carbohydrates throughout the day. Frequent eating keeps insulin high all day. When insulin is high, we cannot burn any of the fat that we have stored on our bodies, so we never go into weight-loss mode. In fact, the more insulin, the more weight we gain. **Managing insulin is a major key to controlling weight.**

We are told that "eat less and exercise more" is the path to weight loss. This does work, but only temporarily. Just eating less of the above diet does not eliminate the cravings. This leaves us with constant hunger. Very few people can keep this up. Also, our body adjusts to the fewer calories eaten, and we simply burn fewer calories, so weight loss stops.

In addition, we have a **"set point"** in weight that our bodies try to keep, so when we lose weight, our bodies try to gain it back. This leads to the typical "yoyo dieting".

When we eat is an important factor in controlling our weight. Leaving time between meals lets our bodies burn ketones instead of glucose. See full discussion later in this chapter.

Eating more healthy fat instead of carbohydrates (keeping our insulin low), combined with leaving more time between meals (letting our bodies burn ketones), is the key to permanent weight loss

without the frequent hunger and cravings.

Let's look at these ideas more closely.

The science behind eating fewer calories

There was a very interesting study done in 1919 at the Carnegie Institute of Washington to test what exactly happens when we reduce calories.[19] Volunteers consumed approximately one third fewer calories than they normally ate. They measured their calories burned while they were eating fewer calories. Their calories burned went from approximately 3,000 to 2,000 per day. What happened? Their metabolism slowed down so that they burned one third fewer calories. **So, 100 years ago, we knew that if we reduce calories, it does not lead to long-term weight loss. It just leads to burning fewer calories to adjust to the fewer calories consumed.**

In 1944, Dr. Ancel Keys performed "the most complete experiment of starvation ever done – the Minnesota Starvation Experiment".[16, 20] Thirty-six young and healthy men were chosen. They had an average weight of 153 pounds. For the first three months, they consumed 3200 calories per day. For the next 6 months, they consumed only 1570 calories. However, the number of calories was adjusted so that they would lose 24 pounds, which was an average of 2.5 pounds per week. Some men had to be limited to 1000 calories per day to lose this much weight. They ate mostly carbohydrates, rarely ate meat or dairy, and walked 22 miles per week as exercise.

After the 6 months of "starvation", they were gradually fed more food until they were again consuming approximately 3,000 calories per day.

What happened when they were in the "starvation" mode?

- Resting metabolic rate dropped by 40%.
- Subjects' strength decreased 21%.
- Heart rate slowed from 55 beats per minute to 35 beats.
- Heart stroke volume decreased by 20%.
- Body temperature dropped to an average of 95.8 degrees F.
- Physical endurance dropped by half.
- Blood pressure dropped.

- They became extremely tired and dizzy.
- They lost hair.
- Their nails became brittle.
- They lost interest in everything except food.
- They had constant hunger. [5]

Their bodies were trying to keep them alive by reducing all caloric expenditures that were not absolutely essential.

Based on the number of calories that were reduced, it would be expected that they would have lost 78 pounds, but they only lost 37 pounds -- less than half of the expected amount. More and more reduction in calories would be required to continue to lose weight.

After they were allowed to eat normally again, they not only went back to their original weight, but they continued to gain.

How long does this reduced metabolism last? A long time. Maybe "indefinitely". [5]

In another study, the National Institute of Health conducted the "most massive, expensive, ambitious and awesome dietary study ever done."[18] They recruited 50,000 post-menopausal women. The experimental group received education sessions, group activities, message campaigns and personalized feedback over one year.

They were told to:

- Reduce fat to 20% of daily calories.
- Eat 5 servings of fruit and vegetables per day.
- Eat 6 servings of grains per day.
- Increase exercise.

The control group was told to eat as they always had, but they were given a copy of the *Dietary Guidelines for Americans*.

The average weight at the beginning of the study was 169 pounds with a BMI of 29.1 (this is almost in the obese range).

The daily calories in the experimental group dropped from 1788 to 1446 per day – **a 342 calorie reduction they maintained over the entire 7 years.**

What else?

- **Fat calories decreased from 38.8 to 29.8.**
- **Carbohydrate increased from 44.5 to 52.7.**

- **Physical activity increased by 14%**

So, what happened to their weight? **If they were eating 342 fewer calories per day, how much might they be expected to lose?**
Let's look at the math:

- There are 3500 calories in a pound.
- If we divide 3500 by 342 (calories reduced per day), we get 10.2.
- Every 10.2 days each woman should lose a pound.
- Over a year (365 days) at a pound every 10.2 days, that comes to about 35.7 pounds in a year.

How much did they lose in the first year? **They lost an average of 4 pounds over the first year, not the 35.7 pounds that might be expected** if calorie reduction were the only factor. During the second year, weight started to go up. **By the end of the 7 years, there was no difference between the experimental and control groups.** This is in spite of the fact that for 7 years, they reduced their caloric intake by 342 calories per day.

So, the "eat less, exercise more" experiment was a total failure.

In summary, we have trouble losing weight with the "eat less, exercise more" system because metabolism slows to match the reduced caloric intake. And metabolism stays low for a very long time.

What else happens when calories are reduced?

Besides metabolism slowing, the other thing that happens is that **we become very hungry. A hormone called ghrelin is produced that stimulates hunger. More hormones are produced that reduce satiety (feeling full). So, caloric reduction leads to being hungrier, and even if you eat, you won't feel as full, so you will want to eat more. "These hormonal changes occur almost immediately and persist almost indefinitely."** [5]

When we lose weight, we feel hungry, cold, tired and depressed. This is how our bodies respond to caloric reduction and weight loss. This makes it even harder to stay on a low-calorie diet. [5]

In summary, the low-calorie, low-fat diet has been proven to fail. Three things happen that make it very difficult to lose weight and keep it off:

- Metabolism slows to match the reduction in calories eaten.
- Hormones are produced by our bodies to increase hunger.
- Hormones are produced by our bodies to keep us from feeling full, so we want to keep eating.

What happens when calories are artificially increased?

Just the opposite happens when people force themselves to eat more than they want to. What happens? Their metabolism speeds up in order to burn up the excess calories.

I thought that the most interesting of these studies was done by Dr. Ethan Sims. [21]It involved convicts at the Vermont State Prison. They were carefully monitored to make sure that they ate 4,000 calories per day, and that physical exercise was strictly controlled.

Just like weight loss, their weight initially rose, then stabilized. Many of them had difficulty continuing to force themselves to keep eating more than their bodies wanted to eat, and some dropped out of the study. However, of those who remained, some were encouraged to eat more than 10,000 calories per day. Over the next 4-6 months, the remaining prisoners did gain up to 25 % of their original body weight. However, it was much less than would be predicted by the additional calories, and there was a huge difference in the amount gained from man to man. These differences could not be understood from caloric intake or exercise.

Their metabolism increased to burn calories faster, increasing so much that they burned 50% more calories, from 1800 calories per day to 2700 calories per day. After the experiment ended, their body weight returned quickly and effortlessly to their original body weight.

This does not seem right, does it? Why did these men not stay fat? So many people in America have gained weight and don't lose it. What is going on here that is so different?

Homeostasis -- our bodies trying to stay at a certain weight

Our bodies have a certain weight that they try to maintain. It is different for all of us.

What determines what that weight is?

- **70% of it is genetic.**
- **That leaves 30% that is under our control.**

How do we know that 70% is genetic?

If we look at a group of adopted kids, do you think they would look like their biological parents or their adoptive parents with regard to weight? It turns out that they look like their biological parents.

Dr. Albert J. Stunkard compared 540 Danish adult adoptees to their biological parents and to their adoptive parents to see which one they resembled with regard to weight. **He found no relationship at all between their adoptive parents and the adult adoptees. However, there was a strong relationship between the adoptees and their biological parents.** [6]

If you take identical twins and put them into different households to be raised, would they look like each other as adults, or like their adoptive parents? They look like each other, not their adoptive parents. Dr. Stunkard examined fraternal and identical twins who were reared apart and together. He determined that 70**% of the tendency to be obese was inherited.** [7]

In other words, 70% of our tendency to be thin or fat is genes. That still leaves 30% under our control.

Our bodies come genetically with a certain idea about how much we should weigh. Some people have thin genes. Some people have genes for larger bodies. Look at your relatives. You probably can get an idea of what genes are in your family.

The 30% under our control

Can we change this set point? Yes.

The reason people gain weight and keep it on, unlike the prisoners described above, is that their set point has been adjusted to a higher level of weight. Why? They have a hormonal imbalance in the body. [3]

Fixing this hormonal imbalance is the key to long-term weight loss. Not eating fewer calories, although calories do matter. Not more exercise, although exercise is good for us for other reasons, and it does burn some additional calories.

We already talked about hormones that increase hunger and reduce satiety. These are powerful hormones in bringing us back to our set point, but they do not change the set point. What changes the set point?

Our set point can be changed by insulin (primarily) and cortisol (secondarily).

Insulin controls weight gain and weight loss

It is well-known that high insulin levels are associated with obesity. However, this does not show causation. It is relatively easy to show that insulin causes weight gain, because of so many diabetics who have regular insulin injections. Many well-controlled studies have shown that **the more insulin that is given, the more the weight that is gained.** [8]

I think a more interesting study is **whether weight would still go up if insulin is increased but calories were decreased**. One study looked at exactly that situation. In a study done in 1993, a group of type 2 diabetic patients were given more and more insulin (from 0 increased to 100, on average) over a period of 6 months while their calories were decreased by 300 per day.

Weight increased by 19 pounds, even though they were eating 300 fewer calories per day! **Increased insulin caused the weight gain, not calories.**

Decreasing insulin causes weight loss.

A study done in 2013 concluded that about **75% of weight loss in obesity can be predicted by insulin levels**. [9]"Obesity is a hormonal, not a caloric imbalance" [5]

How does insulin do this? We are not sure of the exact mechanism. There are many theories. One theory is:

- Eating food, especially carbohydrates, signals the pancreas to make insulin.
- Insulin interacts with each cell to allow the glucose to enter the

cell.

- If we eat a meal, then have a break between meals, insulin spikes, then goes down to its normal low level (good).
- If we eat often throughout the day, we maintain a steady high level of insulin (bad).
- Over time, if we continue with this steady high level of insulin, the cell becomes "insensitive" to insulin and stops allowing the glucose into the cell.
- This may be the beginning of type 2 diabetes.
- If insulin is increased, perhaps through medication, more glucose goes into the cell.
- The cell eventually becomes "insensitive" to this higher amount.
- More and more insulin is needed for the cell to react to the insulin.
- This is called "insulin resistance". [5]

However, for most of us, how insulin does this is not so important. **What matters is "How do we lower insulin levels, lose weight and keep it off (lower our "set point").**

Cortisol also causes weight gain.

Cortisol is the "stress hormone". Under long-term stress, it has the effect of increasing insulin. If increasing cortisol increases insulin, then decreasing cortisol is essential for weight loss.

This is why it is so **important to reduce stress if you are trying to lose weight.** We have been told that calories and exercise (eat less and exercise more) are the keys to losing weight. With this thinking, it is hard to imagine that stress leads to weight gain. But it does. It increases insulin. Insulin controls weight.

There are many ways to decrease stress. There is meditation, exercise, yoga, or changing what we say to ourselves about the events around us.

Most stress is caused by our thoughts. It seems like stress is caused by the things that go on around us, but stress is mostly caused by what we say to ourselves about what goes on around us. This is why some people are very stressed by events while others are not. In order to reduce stress, we need to change our internal dialogue.

Inadequate sleep is a major cause of chronic stress. In 1910, we used to get 9 hours of sleep, on average. Now, more than 30% of adults age 30-64 report getting less than 6 hours of sleep per night. (Bliwise, 1996) **Getting less than 7 hours of sleep seems to be the point where weight gain begins,** with more weight being gained as sleep decreases. [10]

The role of insulin in maintaining weight

The job of insulin is to let energy into the cell.

Normally, what happens when we eat:

- Insulin production is triggered.
- The pancreas releases insulin into the blood.
- Insulin does its job of letting energy into the cell.
- Then insulin goes back down to a normal low level.

But what happens when we eat continuously all day?

- Insulin levels stay high.
- After a while, the cells become used to this high level.
- Cells stop reacting to the insulin.
- They need more and more insulin to notice the increase.
- This creates what is called "insulin resistance".
- This also creates a higher and higher "set point" in weight.

If insulin is controlling our weight, then what we need to do is to lower our insulin production.

What foods increase insulin?

There is an excellent "Insulin Index" chart on Wikipedia. It compares insulin response of food to the glycemic response to food, and it also includes how filling a food is. There is a high correlation between the insulin index and the glycemic index. However, the glycemic index only measures carbohydrates, and the insulin index measures all foods. Fat and protein do not raise blood sugar (glycemic index) because they are not carbs, but they do increase insulin. However, they typically produce a much smaller insulin response than carbohydrates, and, typically, they are more filling. If foods are more filling, we tend to eat less.

Glycemic Index, Insulin index, and Satiety Chart

Food	Glycemic Index (GI) 50 g of carbs	Insulin Index (II) 240 calories	Feeling full (Satiety)
White bread (baseline)	100	100	100
Peanuts	12	20	84
Eggs		31	150
Beef		51	176
Fish		59	225
Apple	50	59	197
Oranges	39	60	202
Brown rice	104	62	132
Doughnuts	63	74	68
Potatoes	141	121	323
Jellybeans	118	160	118

The insulin index is compared to the insulin response to eating white bread. Foods with a low response have low numbers, and foods that trigger a higher insulin response than white bread have a high number.

Discussion of chart

White bread is the food all others are compared to, so it has 100 for every measurement. Note the following:

- **Peanuts** have a low Insulin Index score of 20, but have a fairly good satiety (feeling full) score of 84.
- **Eggs and beef are awesome.** They only trigger insulin 31 and 51, but they are very filling at 150 and 176.
- **Fish are great** with a low insulin score of 59, but extremely filling at 225.

23

- **Apples and oranges** are a surprise with insulin scores of only 59 and 60, but very filling at 197 and 202.
- **Brown rice** has a high glycemic score of 104, but a much lower insulin score at 62, and a fairly high score for being filling at 132. The low carb group often recommends against eating rice because of its high GI, but the insulin score is fairly low, and the satiety score high, so **brown rice looks pretty good on this chart.**
- **Doughnuts** have a lower insulin score than I would have thought (74), but are not very filling, as would be expected. (68)
- **Potatoes** are the big surprise here. We are told by the low-carb people to avoid them because of the high GI of 141, but look how filling they are at **323.** They spike blood sugar, they are moderately high in raising insulin (121), but they are **extremely filling.**
- **Jellybeans** are fairly high at 118 on the GI, get a **whopping 160 for raising insulin** (really bad). However, they are somewhat filling at 118.

What can we conclude from this? Protein and fat do trigger an insulin response, but it is typically much lower than carbohydrates. In addition, fat and protein are both very filling, so we tend to eat less and stay full longer.

If insulin is what controls weight loss and gain, we should be eating fat and protein, and limiting or eliminating foods that spike insulin, such as sugar and flour.

Vegetable oils and inadequate salt can also increase insulin

Eating "vegetable" oils, which create oxidation inside us (bad), and are high in omega 6's (bad), also lead to weight gain independent of the number of calories consumed. [11] (See section on vegetable oils.)

If we don't eat enough salt, our kidneys take the salt out of our blood and recycle it. The kidneys produce cortisol to do this, which increases insulin. (See section on salt.)

Exercise, calories, and weight loss

A woman who weighs 120 pounds typically burns 1500-2000 calories a day, and a man who weighs 180 pounds might burn 2000-2500 calories in a day. There are charts on the internet for a more accurate estimation. Differences are from age, activity level, genetic factors, current weight, and differences in microbiome.

In theory, if you are eating a healthy diet, you should not have to pay any attention to calories. Since your body is getting the nutrition it needs, you should stop being hungry when you have had enough to eat.

There are 3 categories of macronutrients (food with calories). How much does each have?

Carbs: 4 calories per gram
Protein: 4 calories per gram
Fat: 9 calories per gram

What does your body do with these calories?

- **Basic Metabolism.** We use most of our calories to run the basic systems of our bodies. Our brain alone uses about one third of our calories. [12]
- **Digestion.** Another major use of calories is digesting our food.
- **Moving.** We need calories to move our bodies.

What do we normally use our calories for? Almost all of our calories are used to keep our bodies alive, such as breathing, maintaining body temperature, keeping our heart pumping, digesting our food, feeding our brain, liver, kidneys, and repairing our cells. [5] Very little of it is used to fuel "exercise".

In addition, the number of calories we use to keep our bodies alive varies drastically. Reducing calories can decrease our metabolic rate by 40 percent, and increasing calories can increase it by 50%.

Exercise is very important in keeping us healthy, but weight loss is not one of its benefits (or a very minor one). [5]

For a more thorough discussion of these issues, read The *Obesity Code* by Dr. Jason Fung. [5]

(**Personal note:**)

I only burn about 1100 calories per day, in spite of the fact that I exercise about two hours per day. We all have different bodies.

Charts are helpful, but they may not apply to you. I suggest you get to know what your particular body needs. A good beginning is to track what you eat on Cronometer.com. It breaks food down into its various elements (calories, protein, fat, carbs, fiber, vitamins, minerals, etc.). It also tracks exercise and your weight, and many other factors that may be of interest. It's free on the internet.

The role of fiber

One very important role of fiber is to slow down the spiking of blood sugar. This helps keep insulin low. Lower insulin is what we want if we are to keep our weight under control.

Eat a minimum of 25g per day of fiber for women, and 35g for men. Less than 3% of Americans get the minimum recommended intake of fiber.

Why Is Fiber So Important?

A lack of dietary fiber has been associated with a higher risk of diabetes, cardiovascular disease, obesity, and various cancers, as well as higher cholesterol, blood pressure, and blood sugar.

Why aren't Americans eating enough fiber?

Fiber is found only in plants, like beans, fruits, vegetables, and whole grains. Fat and protein have no fiber.

Nearly the entire United States population fails to eat enough whole plant foods. Fiber lowers cholesterol and keeps food moving through our intestines. Eating artificial fiber (fiber pills, etc.) creates gas, so eat real food with fiber.

Vegetables are an excellent source of fiber. Since 80% of your food (by volume) should be vegetables, you will probably get plenty of fiber without thinking about it if you follow my eating plan.

Beans in particular are a great source of protein and fiber. If you are not used to eating beans, try eating just a few every day, then gradually eat more. Your body needs enzymes in the gut to digest beans. As you gradually eat more beans, more enzymes will be made. After you get used to eating beans, the bloating and gas problems should disappear. However, beans are high in carbohydrates, so avoid these if you are on a high fat, low carbohydrate diet.

This is what most researchers say about fiber. However, studies have been done that show we may not need fiber in our diets. People who follow the carnivore diet are not getting any fiber (or very little) and seem to do just fine. [13]

What about the microbiome in our gut? Don't they need fiber?

When you eat may be as important as what you eat – burning ketones

---

A little starvation can really do more for the average sick man
than can the best medicines and the best doctors.
--Mark Twain

All of the cells of our bodies need a steady stream of fuel to keep going. Our bodies are either burning glucose or ketones. After we eat, our bodies make the carbohydrates, and perhaps some proteins in our food, into glucose. This glucose is sent around to all of the cells of our bodies through our blood. After about 8 hours, our bodies have finished burning the glucose. Until we eat again, our bodies begin to burn ketones. These ketones come from stored fat.

However, if we only eat fat, we will continuously burn ketones. It is only carbohydrates and protein that become glucose. Or, if we wait longer between meals, we will burn ketones.

It is vital for our bodies to burn ketones on a regular basis. Why are ketones good for us?

The most important thing they do is:

- They help **clean up the dead or inactive cells in the body so our sick cells can be replaced with healthy ones** This process is called "autophagy", meaning "self-eating".

In addition:

- Ketones **slow the aging process.**
- Ketones **reduce hunger.**
- **Many people lose weight easily when primarily burning ketones.**

- Ketones are the preferred fuel of the body.
- Ketones also help **remove scars.**
- It is important to let our bodies run on ketones occasionally so they can do their job. Cycling through ketosis is our natural state.
- It is good for **curing, or controlling, some diseases, such as diabetes, cancer or epilepsy.**
- Before 1900, the cure for diabetes was eating fat. Fat **does not spike blood sugar.** On a diet of primarily fat, people are burning ketones most of the time.
- **Cancer** thrives on glucose, but most cancers cannot burn ketones, so another way to deal with cancer is to increase ketone production and decrease glucose production.
- Some researchers report that it is insulin insensitivity that creates many of our diseases. Insulin is produced if our cells are using glucose (from carbohydrates). Eating fat and protein also produces insulin, but at a much lower level. Burning ketones rather than glucose allows our bodies to **have a break from high insulin levels.**
- Primitive people did not eat 3 meals a day. They ate when food was available, often not eating every day. We burn ketones when we do not eat (beginning about 8 hours after a meal). Burning ketones frequently is **our natural state.**
- Ketones **improve immune function.**
- They **improve mitochondrial function** (important for energy production).
- **Ketones protect brain function.**
- They **improve inflammation and oxidative stress.** [14] [15]

How do we get our bodies to burn ketones?

Stop eating foods that become glucose

- All carbohydrates, even vegetables, become glucose
- Excess protein becomes glucose
- So, eat only fat, limited protein, and "low carbohydrate" foods, or no carbohydrates at all.
- "Low carbohydrate" usually means 20-50 grams of carbohydrates per day, depending on your body.

- Or don't eat at all (some form of fasting).

Intermittent fasting -- Leaving longer times between eating

- Waiting to have breakfast
- Stop eating in the afternoon or early evening
- This produces a mild ketosis.
- Intermittent fasting can be as short as 10 hours (a 14-hour window of eating in a day) or as long as 22 hours (a 2-hour window for eating in a day).
- 16 hours may be adequate to produce mild ketosis (an 8-hour window of eating)
- Bodies are either burning glucose or ketones
- It burns glucose after we eat (for about 8 hours)
- It burns ketones after food has been digested

Water fasting -- Don't eat anything except water for 3-5 days

- Only do this if you are healthy, not pregnant, and fully grown. This is not for children.
- Taking certain medications may make this impossible.
- To go into full ketosis, it takes about 3 days of not eating any food.
- It is important to drink lots of water while fasting. It helps with hunger and helps with toxin removal.
- Some people experience the "keto-flu". "Keto-flu" is created by too abruptly switching from burning glucose to burning ketones. During ketosis, toxins are released from the stored fat. It is best to start with intermittent fasting to get your body used to burning ketones, and to rid your body of most of the toxins before starting a fast.
- Some people may take vitamins or add a pinch of pink Himalayan salt daily. This helps with hunger and adds minerals. The salt may also help reduce the "keto-flu". [5]

Tips to help when fasting:

- Drink plenty of water. Sometimes hunger is really thirst.
- Stay busy. It takes our minds off hunger.
- Drink coffee, tea, and bone broth. They all help control your appetite.
- Ride the waves of hunger. Hunger is not constant. It comes in

waves. Try drinking liquids until the wave passes.
- Eat nutritious foods on days you are not fasting. Eat lots of healthy fats, and limit or eliminate sugars and carbs. This will make fasting easier.
- Chia seeds will expand if they are soaked in water. They help suppress appetite. This is technically breaking the fast, but "the effect is so light that it does not significantly detract from the benefits of the fast" [16]

Easy way to start fasting: 4 -4 -12

You might want to start with eating 4-4-12. This is at least 4 hours between breakfast and lunch, at least 4 hours between lunch and dinner, and at least 12 hours between dinner and breakfast. This eliminates snacking, and gets your body used to eating fewer meals. This also gives your digestive system a rest between meals. Interestingly, 90% of Americans are not even fasting for 12 hours at night. [17]

After you get used to this, try eliminating breakfast or dinner, so you are only eating two times per day. I have found this to be very easy and painless, once your body gets used to it. This is especially easy if you are eating adequate amounts of fat, and reducing carbs. This helps reduce hunger.

In terms of timing your meals, "scientific literature is clear that the single most important thing you can do is to stop eating at least 3 hours before bedtime." [18]

Does timing meals work even if we are eating junk food?

Absolutely!

Dr. Panda did a number of experiments in humans and rats. I think the most interesting one was a rat study. Rats born to the same mother in the same room were divided into 2 groups. Both groups were fed junk food, high in sugar and carbs, but their eating windows were different. In one group, the food was restricted to an 8-12-hour window. The other group -- fed the same food and the same number of calories -- was given access to the food at all times.

What did they find? "The time-restricted group was protected from obesity, diabetes, cardiovascular disease, systemic inflammation, high cholesterol, and other diseases that the non-time-restricted group fell prey to." [18]

In addition, Dr. Panda found that if he took overweight mice and restricted their eating window to 8-10 hours, he could reverse many of those diseases. He also did a pilot study on humans which showed very promising results. [18]

How long can you live without food?

In 1965 a 27-year-old Scotsman, Angus Barbieri, who weighed 465 pounds decided he was going to fast for one year and live only on his body fat. He was supervised by the Department of Medicine at the Royal Infirmary in Dundee.

He fasted for 1 year and 17 days. He lost 275 pounds, and ended up weighing 180 pounds.

Although he did not eat any food, the hospital staff gave him yeast for the first 10 months and he took multivitamins every day. His potassium got a little low around the 100-day mark, so he was given potassium tablets for about 70 days.

After 5 years he had regained only 16 pounds. [19] [20]

So, with lots of extra body fat, we can live quite a long time without food. Our bodies can stay healthy burning our own body fat.

However, **this is not recommended. It is very risky.** Some people can tolerate this and some people cannot, leading to death from starvation.

I find this story interesting because we have been told that we need to eat small meals all day, or that we need to eat breakfast. This man did just fine by not eating food for over a year.

Body fat is our own personal energy supply that we carry around with us.

(Personal note)

[Intermittent fasting:]

I have been doing intermittent fasting most of my adult life, but not on purpose. I don't like to eat before I exercise, and I am a morning exerciser (swimming, tennis, racquetball, etc.). Also, I am not hungry in the morning. Maybe this is because my body is used to not eating in the morning.

I usually have my first calories about 11 AM. I have a small amount to eat. Then I have one large meal between 2 and 4 PM. I often dance at night, so I usually stop eating about 4 PM. If I eat after that, my stomach is not happy while I am dancing. I have an eating window as small as 2 hours, or as large as 12 hours, but typically about 6 hours. It is not good to drink liquids when eating (dilutes stomach acid), so I do my hydrating before and after meals. This lifetime of intermittent fasting may be one reason why I am so healthy at 72.

> **My opinion regarding ketogenic diets:**

Some people are on a constant low-carbohydrate diet to keep their bodies continuously burning ketones. I have chosen to cycle through burning ketones and burning glucose. On most days I eat high fat and low carbs, and I have occasional days of higher carbohydrates (all real food). Joseph Mercola also recommends occasional days of higher carbohydrates, and discusses the science that supports this. [17]

I do recommend intermittent fasting (time restricted eating). It is not hard or unpleasant to do once your body gets used to it. However, do not do this if you are pregnant, ill, or young (still growing).

For more information about fasting, read *The Complete Guide to Fasting* by Jason Fung [16], *Food* by Mark Hyman [21], or *Fat for Fuel* by Joseph Mercola. [14]

Obesity

"In 1985, not a single American state had a prevalence of obesity above 10 percent. In 2016, the Centers for Disease Control and Prevention (CDC) reported that no state has a prevalence of obesity under 20 percent, and only three states had rates below 25 percent." [22]

--Jason Fung [23]

Based on the total number of obese people in a country, the US ranked #1 in the world with 78 million obese Americans, or 33% of the population. China ranks #2 with 46 million obese people but only 4.4% of the population.

Obesity is an epidemic. Not just in America, but around the world.

How do we measure obesity?

Waist- to-hip ratio. The simplest way to determine your level of being overweight or obese is to measure your hips and waist. If your waist circumference is greater than the widest part of your hips, then you are abdominally obese.

Body Mass Index, or BMI, is another way. Measure your height and weight. Look up a chart in the internet that will tell you what your BMI is. Normal is from 18.5-24.9, 25-29.9 is overweight, and above 30 is obese. This can be somewhat inaccurate because it doesn't differentiate between fat and muscle. If you have very little fat, and a good amount of muscle, the BMI measurement may overestimate your obesity level.

Body fat percent is another way to measure obesity. This is not the same number as Body Mass Index. A woman with a BMI of 20 may have approximately 25% body fat. Experts can measure this, or you can do this the easy way. Look at pictures of people on the internet with different percentages of body fat. For women, obese is over 31%, and for men obese is over 24% (women naturally have more body fat).

Obesity is associated with

- **Cancer.** Thirty-three per cent of cancer deaths are associated with obesity.
- **Hypertension.** But being obese does not mean that you will necessarily have high blood pressure.
- **Type 2 diabetes.**
- **Heart attack.**
- **Stroke.**

However, obesity does not cause these diseases. Most likely, the things that are causing these diseases are also causing weight gain.

Other things associated with obesity.

- **Depression.**
- Having fewer **friends.**
- **Missing more days at work.**
- Having more **health problems.**
- **Energy** issues.
- **Emotional problems.**

- **Sleeping issues**, and sleeping issues contribute to obesity.

Global obesity – a lesson in how to get fat

Globally obesity has exploded.

Populations who continue to eat their indigenous diets typically are very healthy. However, as they change their diets to Western imports, they develop the diseases that are exploding in the developed countries. What exactly are we exporting that has created so much obesity, heart disease, diabetes, etc.? Products with **sugar, vegetable oils, and flour.**

Kellogg's, Kraft, Nestle, McDonalds, Domino Pizza, Coco Cola, Pepsi Cola, all report that their expanding profits are coming from outside North America. [24]

In fact, many companies have more units outside the U.S. than they do within the US. Some examples:

- McDonald's has 14,344 units within the U.S., and 21,914 internationally.
- KFC has only 4,391 in the U.S. but has 15,029 outside the U.S.
- Burger King has just a few more outside the U.S. at 7,246 and 7,126 inside.
- Pizza Hut still has more restaurants inside the U.S. at 7,908 and 7,697 internationally.
- Subway has 26,958 inside the United States, and 16,196 internationally. Subway wins the prize for the most total restaurants at 43,154. [25]

In 1950, there were 100 million obese people around the world, with a world population of 2.52 billion. In 2010, there were 500 million obese people worldwide, with a world population of 6.87 billion. **Obesity had increased 5-fold, while the world population had gone up only 2.7 times.**

America has exported obesity throughout the world. Diabetes, cancer and heart disease accompany this obesity epidemic.

Why has obesity spread around the globe? Countries that are emerging from starvation and poverty now have the money to buy fast food and junk food. They are a new market for American companies.

Companies are not trying to kill everyone. They are in business to make money. However, they are not in the social service business, either. As countries such as Mexico, China, Brazil and India are emerging into the world economy, and a middle class in these countries has more money, these companies are targeting these populations as a new market. [25]

What exactly is going on in these countries?

Mexico

Q: What country gets the prize for the most obese people relative to their population?
A: Mexico.

In 1980, very few people were obese in Mexico. By 2006, two thirds of the adult population was overweight or obese. How did this happen, and so rapidly?!!

Mexicans are getting fatter faster than anywhere else in the world. Why? What changed?

One problem is that the drinking water is not reliable. Instead of drinking water, schools provide soft drinks. "Babies have Coco Cola in their bottles instead of a milk formula."[29]

Companies price soft drinks according to what they think the community can afford. A Coca Cola is cheaper in the small villages than it is in the cities.

Diabetes is now the primary cause of death in Mexico.

China

China went from having very few overweight people in 1990 to one third of adults being overweight on 2006.

Vegetable oils

Part of this is the increased consumption of vegetable oils.

Before WWII the only added fat available was butterfat and lard. Because there was such a shortage of fat during WWII, Japan and America developed a way to extract fats from seeds. This made these vegetable oils abundant and cheap.

These oils, from sesame seeds, cottonseeds, corn, sunflower seeds, and soy beans, have changed the eating habits of the world, including China.

China went from consuming **20 calories a day in oil in the 1980's, to 400 calories a day of vegetable oils.** [24]

Now more than 380 million people in China are overweight or obese.

Sugar

During the 1980's, 2 grams (28.3 grams per ounce) of sugar were consumed per capita in China. This was the lowest in the world at that time. Now the per capita sugar consumption in China is 3.4 pounds [26].

Normally, when eating whole foods, we do not have fat and sugar together. An orange has just sugar, and lots of healthy fiber. A steak has just fat and protein, with no sugar. However, when fat and sugar are combined, such as in ice cream and candy, we love it! And when flour is added, Wow! We find it very hard to resist such foods as cookies, cakes, pies, and doughnuts.

Brazil

Each year, the obesity rate in Brazil goes up 1 per cent. In 2006, 50% of adults were obese. [24]

What changed here?

Before the 1990's, most people in Latin America got their food from local farmer's markets. Now the supermarkets dominate food sales. In 1990 people in Latin America bought only 15% of their food from a supermarket. By 2000 it was 60%. In 10 years, that is a huge change! Food is more reliably sanitary, and the cheap processed foods are abundantly available in these supermarkets. The 1990's is when obesity began to explode in Latin America. [24]

American companies are making the world fat with their cheap exports of processed foods.

Let's look at Nestles. They have special products for Latin America. They sell smaller packages that make for cheap snacks. They add vitamins to some products so they can sell them as "health foods".

However, even though the foods are cheap, obesity-related illness costs the Brazilian health system around $2.1 billion per year. [24]

India

Obesity used to be rare in India. Not anymore.

Indians used to eat locally grown foods that were cooked at home. Now most meals are eaten out, and much of it is "junk foods" that are high in calories and low in nutrition.

Indians tend to get diabetes at a younger age than Westerners, which means that they are less effective in what should be the most productive years of their lives. [24]

Is obesity causing diabetes?

- Obesity is increasing worldwide by 2.78% per year 1975-2015. [27]
- Diabetes is increasing worldwide by 4.07% per year 1980-2014. [28] [29]

Note that diabetes is going up faster than obesity. If obesity caused diabetes, how could this be true?

Let's look at the 240 million adults in the U.S. Thirty per cent are obese (72 million), and 70% are normal weight (168 million). Eighty per cent of the obese are sick. It might look like obesity is causing illnesses. However, 20% are healthy.

Guess what? Forty per cent of people who are normal weight are sick. There are actually more sick people in the normal weight group (67 million) than in the obese group (57 million). Why? Because there are more of them. [29]

Obesity is associated with many diseases, but it does not cause them. It is a symptom. Something else is causing diseases. What is actually causing these diseases? Sugar, flour and seed oils, the main ingredients of processed foods.

Interesting fact: For people who seem to be unable to lose weight any other way, a high fat diet is recommended, maybe even only fats for a period of time. They lose weight. I'm not recommending a 100% fat diet, but it is interesting to know.

Personal Note

I traveled by train from the southern tip of India to New Delhi in 1974. I was told by other Westerners to not drink the water or eat any food in the train stations. They said to drink only American Coca-Colas and eat only hard-boiled eggs. That is what I did for the 3 days it took to reach New Delhi.

My American friend got too hungry to do this, so he got out and ate in the train stations. A few weeks later, he became very ill with hepatitis.

In spite of the sugar and chemicals in Coca-Cola, it may sometimes be a better choice than the local drinking water. I think that is one reason why the locals drink Coca-Colas and put it in their babies' bottles, and why they eat packaged foods. Short-term, they don't get diarrhea, dysentery, hepatitis, etc. from unsanitary food and contaminated water. Long-term, they may become obese, have diabetes, or heart disease. As unhealthy as sodas are, they may be safer than drinking the local water and eating the unpackaged foods.

However, we in America don't have to make that choice. Almost all food is sanitary and disease-free. We are choosing unhealthy foods because of convenience, habit, and cost.

The things that are creating global obesity are the same things that are creating obesity here in America. These are sugar, flour, and vegetable oils. Avoid these and you will be much healthier.

$$\boxed{\text{Personal Note}}$$

$$\boxed{\textbf{Controlling my weight}}$$

As I stated in the opening of this chapter, doing the research for this chapter helped me to have total control over my weight for the first time in my life.

I was already doing many of the things I cover in this book. I had largely eliminated added sugars and grains, added more healthy fats, ate adequate healthy protein, and ate only real food, mostly organic. In addition, I was typically fasting for 18 hours per day (only eating within a 6-hour window per day). However, I still struggled to control my weight.

My normal lifetime weight is about 125. Sometimes it goes up to about 135. I know that does not sound like much, but it was for me. When I did gain weight, it seemed that I was almost powerless to stop it, and I did not know why I was gaining weight.

After doing the research for this chapter, it became clear that if increased insulin leads to weight gain, it is logical that I should decrease my insulin. It is difficult for individuals to test insulin, but is easy to test blood sugar. These are not the same, but they often go up and down together.

I decided to test my blood sugar throughout the day. Blood sugar testing kits are cheap and easy to use, and are probably for sale in your local drug store.

Every morning my blood sugar was about 85. I often had hot chocolate in the morning with one cup of whole milk, water, and cacao powder. After I drank this, my blood sugar was about 125. I think it was the lactose (sugar) in the milk that was triggering the increase in blood sugar. The rest of the day, my blood sugar was usually 90-100.

I also tracked what I ate on cronometer.com, a free website. I knew that a major source of carbs in my day was from the milk in my hot chocolate. The next highest source was fresh fruit. This app also tracks net carbs. Net carbs are the carbs with the fiber taken out.

My net carbohydrates for the day were typically about 50. I eliminated milk and fruit, and anything else that had very many carbs. Now my blood sugar stayed between 82 and 105 all day, and my net carbohydrates were about 20. I still ate primarily non-starchy vegetables. These have carbs, but not that many. I also ate heathy fats and protein.

I lost 3 pounds in the first few days, and then I stopped losing.

I dropped my net carbs to under 10, and I started losing weight again, and without hunger! I kept eating my usual number of calories, but occasionally lowered the calories because I wasn't very hungry. The amazing thing is that lowering carbs almost eliminates hunger. Who knew?

What did I eat? For me, it wasn't much of a change. No milk, no fruit, more meat with fat, only vegetables on the "very low carbs" list, cooked in lots of fat (butter, coconut oil, or bacon fat).

Quite honestly, I was shocked that this worked. After a lifetime of fighting my weight, I finally had control. And it was so easy! Wow!

One thing that made it easier to keep my net carbs low was eating a few chocolate fat bombs. They are very filling. See recipe section.

Usually, losing weight means deprivaton and pain. Deprivation from not eating yummy foods, and pain in the form of constant hunger. Losing weight by reducing carbs, for me, was neither of these things. I wasn't hungry, and I ate my favorite yummy foods. Again, wow!

Take away:

- "Eat less and exercise more" is not a successful strategy for weight loss over time.
- It turns out that insulin, and secondarily cortisol, are the hormones that we need to focus on if we want to maintain a lifetime of health and ideal weight. Insulin is controlled primarily by what and when we eat. Cortisol is controlled primarily by stress. We have control over both of these.
- It is very difficult to fight our hunger. However, if we can lower our hunger through lowering insulin levels, our bodies, on their own, should want less food, maintain a steady metabolism, lower its set point of weight, and lose weight.
- Leaving more time between meals is an important part of controlling our weight.
- As countries add processed foods to their diets that contain sugar, flour, and vegetable oils, they began gaining weight, leading to an obesity epidemic around the world. It is clear, from watching this happen, that these are the foods that cause obesity and chronic diseases.
- To lose weight, lower your "set point", and experience only normal hunger, the key is to reduce insulin, and keep cortisol low. So, eat non-starchy vegetables, aviod foods high in carbohydrates, eat adequate protein and healthy fats, let your body have a break from eating (from 8-22 hours per day), and keep stress under control.
- Bottom line on controling weight: Eating carbs increases insulin. The more insulin, the more weight gain. Decreasing carbs lowers the insulin level, lowers hunger, which leads to less weight gain, or weight loss if insulin is low enough. Just reducing calories leads to initial weight loss, then the metabolism slows down and hunger is increased, so weight loss stops, and often the weight comes right back on.

Chapter 3

Macronutrients

Macronutrients are the three food groups that contain calories: fat, carbohydrate, and protein.

Health experts have been arguing for years over how much of each one is healthy. Let's look at what research tells us.

Macronutrient #1: Fats

"The evidence in support of eating fats – traditional, unrefined fats from plants and animals – is overwhelming. The largest randomized controlled study comparing a high-fat diet to a low-fat diet, the PRE-DIMED study, showed that a high-fat diet reduces heart disease, diabetes, and obesity. We need fats for healthy cell membranes. We need them to make hormones (like testosterone and estrogen) and immune cells, to regulate inflammation and metabolism. We need fats because 60 percent of our brains are fat. That sounds pretty important, doesn't it?"

--Dr. Mark Hyman [21]

This section on fat covers:

- **Are fats healthy?**

- **Are saturated fats healthy?**
- **What causes heart disease and strokes?**
- **Is high cholesterol the problem?**
- **Is high LDL the problem?**
- **Some thoughts about statins**

Are fats healthy?

Some things to consider:

- The human brain is nearly 60 percent fat
- Essential Fatty Acids (EFA) are crucial for our brain health.
- We can't make them. We have to get them from our food.
- Before modern medications, epilepsy and diabetes were treated by eating more fat because fat does not spike blood sugar.

Healthy fats (some controversy about the animal fats)

- avocado
- coconut oil (great for cooking)
- olive oil
- wild caught Alaskan salmon (for omega 3 fatty acids)
- gouda cheese (for K2)
- pasture-fed or grass-fed animal products (for K2 and healthy fats) with no pesticides, hormones, or antibiotics

Unhealthy fats

- Processed vegetable oils such as corn oil, soybean oil, cottonseed oil, any hydrogenated or partially hydrogenated oil, margarine, canola oil, rapeseed oil, grapeseed oil, sunflower oil, safflower oil, and rice bran oil
- Trans fats
- Fried foods
- Conventionally raised animals fed corn and soy (too many omega 6's, and poison in the form of glyphosate), and given hormones and antibiotics. This is most of the meat in the grocery store.

Does eating fat make you fat

- People with high fat diets eat fewer calories and usually lose weight
- Fat does have calories, and if you eat too much, you will gain weight, but no more than eating too much of any food.
- We need fat in our diet to stay healthy (some disagreement about this).
- Some vitamins are fat-soluble. These are D3, K2, E, and A. We need to eat them with fat in order for our bodies to use them.
- Omega-3 fatty acids (found in salmon, nuts and seeds) are very good for our health.
- Fat helps us feel full.
- We need fats for healthy cell membranes. [21]

Healthy fats

There is a debate among food experts. Some say that we were completely wrong about saturated fats and it is safe to eat as much as we want [14]. Others tell us to eat no animal products at all [30]. Some say a limited amount is fine [1]. This list is what I believe is healthy, based on research.

- **Meat.** Cattle raised the conventional way (taken to feed lots at the end of their lives to fatten them up) should be avoided because of the high amounts of omega 6 from eating grains instead of grass, the added hormones, use of antibiotics, and the level of poison residue (glyphosate from GMO corn and soy). **Grass-fed beef, pasture fed chickens and organic pork are considered healthy to eat, with no added hormones, and no antibiotics.** What about **bacon**? Before 1900, the primary cooking oil was lard (fat from pork). Heart attacks and cancer were rare compared to today. **Buy bacon that is uncured, no added nitrates or nitrites, no antibiotics or hormones, and organic.** I believe that lard and coconut oil are ideal for cooking.
- **Milk and milk products.** Organic pasture-fed dairy is healthy. Avoid other dairy (fed GMO corn and soy with glyphosate residue, or with added hormones and antibiotics) Seventy-five per cent of the world has trouble digesting lactose, so milk may

not be a good choice for these people (see chapter on what your ancestors ate).[35]

- **Full-Fat Yogurt** has healthy fats, and probiotic bacteria. Do not eat yogurt with added sugar.
- **Sour cream and cream cheese** are healthy if they are from grass-fed cows. However, they are high in calories, so should be eaten sparingly.
- **Cheese** is a great source of calcium, vitamin B12, phosphorus and selenium, and contains all sorts of other nutrients. It is also very rich in protein. It is best to eat cheese from pasture-fed cows in part for the K2. In addition, the bacteria that make gouda and brie also have K2. [31] However, other cheeses have healthy fat and protein, but they are high in calories, so eat sparingly. One ounce is plenty.
- **Whole eggs** are loaded with vitamins and minerals. Be sure to eat eggs from pasture-fed chickens. You get the extra bonus of Vitamin K2 and D3. And eat the whole egg, not just the whites.
- **Fatty Fish.** I recommend wild Alaskan Sockeye salmon. It's great for omega 3 fatty acids, and has less mercury contamination than most other fish. See fish section under protein for more information.
- **Dark Chocolate** is 11% fiber and contains over 50% of the RDA for iron, magnesium, copper and manganese. It is also loaded with antioxidants. Just make sure to choose quality dark chocolate, with at least 70% cocoa. I prefer cacao, a less processed version of cocoa. Cacao also tastes better. I make my own "chocolate fat bombs" so I can control the amount of sweetener (see recipe section).
- **Avocados** are a great source of fat, magnesium, potassium, and fiber.
- **Nuts and seeds** have fats, fiber and protein. Nuts are also high in vitamin E and loaded with magnesium. Studies show that people who eat nuts tend to be healthier, and have a lower risk of obesity, heart disease, and type 2 diabetes. Almonds, pecans, cashews, pumpkin seeds, and hemp seeds are excellent choices. Chia Seeds have omega-3's, are packed with fiber, minerals and are anti-inflammatory. Flax seeds have lots of omega 3 fatty acids, but we cannot digest them as whole seeds. They need to be made into flour or ground before eating. Seeds go bad quickly, so store them in the refrigerator or freezer.

- **Coconut Oil** is an excellent oil to cook with. It does not oxidize when heated like many other oils do.

Should you eat more fat? If these apply to you, try increasing your fat intake.

- You are hungry even though you have eaten adequate amounts of food.
- You are often cold.
- You skin is dry.
- You have problems concentrating, or are often tired.

What are the different kinds of fats?

Keep in mind that most fats are a mix. For example, one tablespoon of butter is mostly saturated fat at 7.2 g of saturated fat, but butter also has 3g of monounsaturated fat, and .4g of polyunsaturated fat. Lard (pig fat) is 5g of saturated fat, 5.8g of monounsaturated fat, and 1.4g of polyunsaturated fat. Even though lard is an animal fat, it has more monounsaturated fat than saturated fat. Even olive oil has some saturated fat at 1.9g, but is mostly monounsaturated fat at 9.9g, with 1.4g of polyunsaturated fat per tablespoon. [32]

The following list is the primary component of each oil.

Saturated fats in animal products (healthy)

- Dairy (butter, cheese, milk, cream, sour cream, yogurt)
- Eggs
- Meat

Saturated fats in vegetable products (healthy)

- Coconut oil
- Cocoa butter

Unsaturated fats:

Unsaturated fats are divided into 2 groups: Monounsaturated fats and polyunsaturated fats. These are:

Monounsaturated fats (healthy)

- Olive oil
- Lard (pig fat)

Polyunsaturated fats high in omega 3's (healthy)

These are really good for us, and help to balance out having too many omega 6's.

- Fish oils
- Flaxseeds

Polyunsaturated fats high in omega 6's (unhealthy)

Do not eat these. These are often found in packaged foods.

- Corn oil
- Cottonseed oil
- Canola oil
- Safflower oil
- Soybean oil
- Rapeseed oil

- Grapeseed oil

Saturated Fat -- good or bad?

The truth about saturated animal fat:

- Eating saturated fats can raise blood cholesterol. That part is true for some people.
- However, eating saturated fat instead of foods high in carbohydrates, tends to change your LDL cholesterol from the small LDL (bad LDL) to the large fluffy kind of LDL (harmless LDL). The type of LDL you have is far more important than the number of LDL particles. [33]
- The amount of cholesterol in your blood is largely regulated by your liver, not your diet.
- Saturated fat raises HDL cholesterol (good). [33] **HDL cholesterol (high is good) is a much better indicator of future heart health than LDL cholesterol.**

- Several studies show that eating saturated fat does not increase heart disease. For example, a study from Harvard concluded that eating more saturated fat is "associated with less progression of coronary atherosclerosis, whereas carbohydrate intake is associated with a greater progression." [34]
- The Nurses' Health Study found that refined carbohydrates were shown to be associated with an increased risk of coronary heart disease.
- **The balance between omega-6 fats (found in vegetable oils), and omega-3 fats (found in nuts, flaxseeds, fish, and grass-fed meat) is far more important than saturated fat intake is.** This should be a one-to one ratio. For many Americans, the ratio maybe as high 25 to 1 (too many Omega-6's).
- Low-fat diets work because they reduce omega-6 fats (often in processed foods), not because they reduce saturated fat. [33]

Saturated fats and coronary heart disease

Eating saturated fats can raise total cholesterol. That is true. However, the real question is whether or not eating saturated fat causes heart disease. Otherwise, high cholesterol does not matter. So, does eating saturated fat cause heart disease?

A **meta-analysis** is a study that reviews many other studies to see if there are trends, or conclusion that can be drawn from a much larger sample size (all of the studies combined). They exclude all of the studies that are poorly done, and combine the rest into one large group.

One group looked at the relationship between eating saturated fat and coronary heart disease (CHD), stroke or cardiovascular disease (CVD). [35]

Twenty-one studies were included in the meta-analysis, with a total of 347,747 subjects. They were followed for between 5 and 23 years.

Did eating saturated fat increase their risk of CHD or stroke? No.

Those who ate the most saturated fat had the same rate of CHD, stroke and CVD as those who ate the least amount of saturated fat.

Another meta-analysis done in 2011 published in the *Netherlands Journal of Medicine* found the same thing.

The authors conclude, "The dietary intake of saturated fatty acids is associated with a modest increase in serum total cholesterol, but not associated with cardiovascular disease." [36]

Again, eating saturated fats does not increase heart disease.

Total cholesterol and coronary heart disease

Researchers in Japan performed another meta-analysis involving more than 150,000 people who were followed for about 5 years. They put people into **4 categories based on their cholesterol levels:**

- Less than 160 mg/dl
- 160 to 199 mg/dl
- 200to 239 mg/dl
- Higher than 240 mg/dl

Q: Which group should die at a highest rate?

We have been told that the higher your cholesterol, the more likely you are to die. Right?

Well, just the opposite turned out to be true.

A: The group with the lowest cholesterol level died at the highest rate. This isn't just cardiac events, but all-cause mortality.

So, the higher your cholesterol, the less likely you are to die for any reason.

The best study on saturated fat and heart health

The A TO Z Weight Loss Study is the best study ever done on the effect of eating high-fat, high saturated-fat diets on weight and on risk factors for both heart disease and diabetes. [37]

There were 4 groups:

- **The Atkins diet (A):** Only 20 grams of carbs for the first few months, then up to 50 grams of carbs. Unlimited animal fats and protein.
- **Traditional diet (T):** Calories are restricted, carbs 55-60% of calories, fat less than 30%, saturated fat limited to 10%, and exercise was encouraged.
- **The Ornish diet (O):** Fewer than 10% of calories from fat, with

meditation and exercise.
- **The Zone diet (Z):** 30% of calories from protein, 40% from carbs, and 30% from fat.

What were the results? For those who ate the most fat and protein:

- **Their risk of having a heart attack decreased significantly.**
- They lost as much weight or more than the others.
- HDL cholesterol went up (good).
- Triglycerides went down (good).
- Blood pressure went down (good).
- Their total cholesterol didn't change much.
- Their LDL cholesterol went up slightly, but it was the large fluffy kind (harmless) not the small dense kind (deadly).

Christopher Garner, director of Nutrition Studies at the Stanford Prevention Research Center, had been a vegetarian for 25 years before he did this study. **He did the study because he was concerned that a diet like Atkins, high in meat and saturated fats, was dangerous. He called the results "a bitter pill to swallow".** [37]

The case for eating animal fats

French Paradox

If you are still convinced that eating fat kills people, consider the "French paradox". The French consume some of the highest fat diets in the world, especially saturated fats. They are famous for their butter and cream sauces. In spite of this, they have almost the lowest heart attack rate in the world. At least, this was true until they started eating more like Americans.

If eating fat, especially saturated fats, killed people, the French could not have such a low rate of heart disease.

The Eskimos

In the early 1900's, Vilhjalmur Stefansson lived with a group of Eskimos (the Copper Inuit) who had been quite isolated from the rest of civilization. Stefansson spent a total of 11 years living as "an Eskimo among Eskimos". [38]

The view was then, as it is now, that the less meat you ate, the healthier you would be.

However, he found something quite different to be true. The Copper Inuit **lived almost exclusively on fat, meat, and fish**. What exactly did they eat? "For six to nine months they ate nothing but caribou, followed by months of exclusively salmon, and a month of eggs in the spring. Observers estimated that some 70 to 80 percent of the calories in their diet came from fat." [39]

Notice what parts of the animal they prized:

- The fat deposits behind the caribou eye
- Fat along the jaw
- The rest of the head
- The heart
- The kidney
- The shoulder

What about the muscle meat (the part that we prize)?

· "The leaner parts, including the tenderloin, they fed to the dogs." [40]

According to the thinking of the day, as now, these people should have had massive heart disease. But what did he find?

High blood pressure, heart disease and stroke were virtually unknown, and they seldom suffered from cancer. He also never saw a fat Eskimo.

These were not genetic traits. As soon as the Eskimos started eating standard Western food, they became fat and developed the same diseases that the rest of Americans have.

After living many years with the Inuit, Stefansson came back to New York. In 1928, he and a colleague agreed to eat nothing but meat and water for an entire year. They started out in Bellevue Hospital where they were closely supervised for the first few weeks, then they went home to finish the year.

The thinking of the day was that they would die on such a diet. He and his friend did not die. In fact, they thrived. At the end of a year, the scientists who were on his medical team could find nothing wrong with either of them. The only time he got sick is when he was encouraged to eat only lean meat. When he added the fat again, he became healthy.

Why didn't they get scurvy? They ate the whole animal, including the bones, liver, and brain, which contain vitamin C. They got calcium from chewing on the bones, just as the Eskimos did.

Stefansson continued this diet for most of his life. He did go off the diet for a period of time. He gained weight and became quite grumpy, according to his wife. [40]

When he went back on the meat and fat diet, he lost the weight, and became his usual happy self again. He died at eighty-three.

The Maasai

The Maasai are a tribe in Kenya. **The men are known for eating only meat, milk, and blood.** They would sometimes mix the milk with cow's blood. They also ate lamb, goats, and beef. They would sometimes eat 4 to 10 pounds of fatty beef per person. Animal fat was 66 per cent of their calories, which means that it was primarily saturated fat. For men in the warrior class, no vegetables were eaten. [41]

They drink 3-5 quarts of raw whole milk per day. They consume 3,000 calories per day.

They are very lean and healthy people. The men weigh an average of 128 pounds.

Interestingly, on this diet, their blood pressure was 50% lower than Americans at that time, and their blood pressure did not increase with age. [41]

What about heart attacks?

George V. Mann studied the Maasai in the early 1960's and could find almost no heart disease at all. He did electrocardiograms on 400 men. He did autopsies on fifty Maasai men, and found only one who seemed to have had a heart attack. [41]

They also showed no evidence of cancer or diabetes.

How could this be true if a high cholesterol diet (high in animal fats) causes heart attacks?

In spite of this clear information, the American Heart Association says we should eat no more than 5-6% saturated fat.

Again, the Maasai warriors consume a diet of 66% saturated fat with no heart disease.

Yes, the Maasai were in great health on an animal diet, but how long did they live? There does not seem to be clear information about this. So, let's look at another example of primarily meat-eaters right here in America.

American Indians

The Native Americans of the Southwest were studied between 1898 and 1905 by Ales Hrdlicka. **These Native Americans ate a diet primarily of meat, mostly buffalo.** On this diet, they were extremely healthy and lived to a surprisingly old age. [42]

He examined two thousand Native Americans and found:

- Only three cases of heart disease
- No atherosclerosis (plaque in the arteries)
- Varicose veins were rare
- No appendicitis
- No ulcers of the stomach
- No liver diseases
- No cancer
- No peritonitis (inflammation of the silk-like membrane that lines your inner abdominal wall and covers the organs within your abdomen) [43]

So, we can conclude that eating primarily meat does not cause these diseases. But what about longevity?

According to the 1900 US Census, how many Native Americans lived to 100 or older?

- 224 per million men
- 254 per million women

At the same time, in the white population, how many lived to 100 or older?

- 3 per million men
- 6 per million women

So, here is a population eating primarily meat with both spectacularly good health and impressive longevity.

There are many other examples throughout the world. In isolated populations that still ate their original diet, there were many reports of indigenous cultures being free of the diseases that have come to be so common in the western world.

For example, George Prentice, wrote in 1923 about the inhabitants of Southern Central Africa:

"The negroes, when they can get it, eat far more meat than the white people. There is no limit to the variety or the condition, and some might wonder whether there is a limit to the quantity. They are only vegetarians when there is nothing else to be had . . . Anything from a fieldmouse to an elephant is welcomed." [39]

The developed world has been on a high carbohydrate/low fat diet for at least 50 years. How is that working?

- In Britain fat consumption has been stable since 1910, while the number of heart attacks has increased 10 times between 1930 and 1970. **So, in Britain, something is causing more heart attacks, but it is not eating fat.**
- Since WWII the Japanese have been eating more and more animal fat, while fewer and fewer of them die from heart attacks. In addition, mortality from most diseases decreased in Japan as they at more animal fat.
- In Switzerland, after WWII, as the intake of animal fat went up by 20%, the death rate from heart disease steadily went down. **So, in Switzerland, eating more fat is correlated with lower heart disease.**
- In the USA, between 1930 and 1960, mortality from heart disease increased 10 times, while the consumption of animal fat decreased. **Again, in the US, there is a negative correlation between eating fat and heart disease.**
- In Yugoslavia, between 1955 and 1965, the number of heart attacks increased 10 times, while fat intake went down by 25%. **Again, in Yugoslavia, as eating fat goes down, heart attacks go up.** [44]

This is exactly the opposite of what we have been told. As we eat more animal fat, heart attacks go down. As we eat less animal fat, heart attacks go up. In fact, dying from all causes goes down as we eat more fat.

Study after study shows these same results, yet conventional medicine is still trying to lower cholesterol by limiting the consumption of animal fats, and by taking medication (primarily statins).

Are there unhealthy fats that we should avoid eating?

Yes. We should avoid eating seed and bean oils, such as canola oil, cottonseed oil, soybean oil, and corn oil.

Coconut oil, olive oil, and avocado oil are healthy vegetable oils to eat.

See chapter on oils for a more thorough discussion.

I recommend the book, *The big Fat Surprise Why Butter, Meat & Cheese Belong in a Healthy Diet*, by Nina Teicholz, for a more thorough review of these issues.

What about vegans and vegetarians?

We have probably all **heard that vegetarians are supposed to be healthier than meat-eaters**. In the longest observational study on vegetarians, 63,550 middle-aged European men and women were followed for a decade. They found **no difference in mortality between vegetarians and non-vegetarians.** [45]

Mark Hyman thinks that the "healthy user effect" is why vegans and vegetarians do as well or better than meat-eaters in some studies.

- Vegetarians on the whole are more health conscious and more likely to exercise and to avoid junk foods, sugar, processed foods, and smoking. They even floss their teeth more.
- Meat eaters tend to have worse habits.
- Studies that compare health-conscious meat eaters with vegetarians show no difference in health outcomes. [46]

Vegetarians often choose this lifestyle because they do not want to do harm to living creatures. Lierre Keith has an interesting viewpoint on this. In *The Vegetarian Myth* [47] Keith says that:

- The plowing of fields, clearing of forests, and growing of plants requires the **wholesale destruction of entire ecosystems.**
- This includes the death of birds, rodents, bugs, worms, and trillions of microbes in the soil.
- **Agriculture is the most destructive thing humans have done to the planet.**
- For most of human history browsers and grazers ate what we could not eat -- cellulose, and turned it into what we could eat -- protein and fat.
- Cattle should still be eating grasses. However, we now feed them grain. This is unhealthy for the animals, unhealthy for the soil and environment, and unhealthy for the people eating it.

- Sheep and goats should never eat grain.
- Chickens get fatty liver disease if fed grain exclusively.
- 98% of the American prairie is gone, turned into a monocrop of grains.
- **The disappearance of topsoil is as much of a threat as global warming.**
- **No matter what you eat, something has to die to feed you.**

There is an excellent TedTalk on this subject given by Brian Sanders. [48]

Vegans and vegetarians may be eating animal products without realizing it. The soil that grows vegetables often has animal products added, such as bone meal and oyster shells, so it will be healthy enough to grow vegetables. [46]

It is possible to be healthy on a vegan or vegetarian diet, but it is harder to get adequate nutrition. Eat enough healthy fats (nuts, seeds, avocados, etc.) and avoid sugar and processed foods.

I support anyone's choices of food. I know that many people choose to avoid animal products for moral, health or environmental reasons. In addition, everyone has a different body. Do what works for you. [46]

However, these are things that might be useful to know when making your food choices.

The true cause of heart disease

What we have been told about the cause of heart disease:

Fat has been unfairly demonized over the last 50 years. We have all heard that eating saturated animal fats raises our cholesterol, and high cholesterol clogs our arteries. Too much cholesterol leads to heart attacks and strokes, and therefore eating saturated animal fats should be eliminated. This was the theory that gained popular support.

However, it happens to be wrong. So, what is the truth about saturated animal fat, cholesterol, and heart disease?

Plaque does build up in our arteries, but it is not from eating saturated fat. Plaque builds up because of inflammation.

- Eating high glycemic foods, such as sugar and white flour, creates inflammation. This irritates the walls of the arteries.

- Cholesterol acts like a band aid to help heal the damaged artery walls.
- This does create plaque building up on the artery walls (which is bad).
- Pieces of plaque can break off, travel down the artery and block the flow of blood.
- If that blockage is in the heart, it is a heart attack.
- If that blockage is in the brain, it is a stroke.
- It can also happen in other parts of the body. [33]

What foods cause inflammation?

- **Fried foods** (many oils become oxidized when heated). They turn into very unhealthy fats.
- **Most vegetable oils** (margarine, butter replacements, hydrogenated oils, artificial fats, soybean oil, canola oil, cottonseed oil, and other seed and bean oils.)
- **White sugar and wheat flour** (anything that spikes blood glucose)
- **Most processed and packaged foods** if they are made with the above ingredients.

So, eat fewer omega 6 fatty acids, and fewer foods that increase insulin. See chapter on reversing diseases for a longer explanation.

Interesting cholesterol facts:

- Around 25 percent of all body cholesterol is in the brain.
- People who live the longest tend to have high cholesterol.
- Statins (to lower cholesterol) are one of the world's most prescribed medicines. They make billions for drug companies. Most of the research on statins is sponsored by the drug companies.
- Research that is not sponsored by the drug companies shows that high cholesterol levels are correlated with living longer
- A high-fat diet – saturated or otherwise – is not correlated with heart disease, except for the unhealthy seed and bean oils, often called "vegetable oils".

Cholesterol is primarily made in the liver. If we need more, it makes more. If we have enough, it makes less.

Cholesterol is responsible for:

- **Making estrogen, progesterone, testosterone, cortisone, and other vital hormones.**
- Making **Vitamin D.**
- Making **bile acids.** Bile is needed to absorb fat-soluble vitamins (vitamin D, A, K, and E). We cannot live without these vitamins. [49]
- It is instrumental in **fighting toxins.**
- You need cholesterol to **make brain cells and for memory.** Around 25% of all cholesterol is used by the brain.
- **Synapse formation** is dependent on cholesterol. Our brain and nervous system depend on the transmission of electrical or chemical messages from one nerve cell to another. The area between these cells that carries this message is called a synapse. We need properly functioning synapses to learn and form memories. This is why one of the effects of a statin drug (which reduces the body's ability to make cholesterol) is loss of brain function. [50]
- A major part of our brain and spinal cord is a fatty substance called **myelin.** It coats the cells like the covering around an electrical wire. Myelin provides insulation and nourishment for the cells. About 20% of our brain and spinal cord is made up of myelin. [51] When myelin is not doing its job, multiple sclerosis (MS) develops. Interfering with cholesterol production also interferes with myelin production.
- Cholesterol is essential for the **developing brain and eyes of the fetus and newborn.** [52] Breast milk supplies this cholesterol.
- Sadly, most infant formulas follow the anti-cholesterol dogma and provide almost no cholesterol in their products.

Bottom line, you cannot live without cholesterol. [44]

Is LDL causing heart disease?

The Isehara Study was conducted in Japan in a city with a population of about 100,000. The researchers looked at medical records of 8,340 men (average age 64) and 13,591 women (average age 61) and divided them into 7 groups of LDL levels.

In both groups, overall mortality was highest in the group with the lowest LDL levels (less than 80). However, men in the group with the highest LDL levels (greater than 180) died more from heart disease, but because the all-cause mortality was lower, even in this group high LDL led to fewer deaths. Interestingly, fewer women died from heart disease in the group with the highest LDL levels.

In summary, both men and women lived longer with the highest LDL, although high LDL levels are even better for women than for men. This is exactly the opposite of what we have been told.

Low cholesterol is bad

- Low cholesterol (160 or less) has been linked to **depression, aggression, cerebral hemorrhages, and loss of sex drive.**
- Lowering cholesterol is associated with **deaths** that are unrelated to heart disease. These include cancer, suicide, violence, and accidents. [44]
- Low cholesterol is associated with **brain hemorrhage and stroke.** [53], [54]
- People with low cholesterol are more likely to get **infections,** have them longer, and even more likely to die of infections. [53]

High Cholesterol is actually good

- **People who live the longest have high cholesterol.** [44]
- High cholesterol protects us from infections, strokes, heart disease, and many other health problems. [53]

More important than cholesterol numbers are cholesterol ratios:

- HDL/cholesterol ratio should be above 24%.
- Triglyceride/HDL ratio should be below 2. [55]
- Triglycerides are in part a function of the amount of sugar you are eating. If your triglycerides are too high, try eating less sugar and other foods that spike blood sugar. [33]

Other studies show that eating saturated fats does raise cholesterol

But eating saturated fats also raises HDL (the good cholesterol) and the good kind of LDL (the large, fluffy kind).

Actually, low HDL is the best predictor of heart disease, not LDL. More on this later.

Research does not support a direct relationship between eating saturated fat and heart disease.

Remember, it is the ratio that matters.

How does cholesterol impact longevity?

Are there any commonalities among centenarians in their blood work? In 1992, a group of researchers looked at exactly that. [56]

What do people who live over 100 have in common?

- **Low triglycerides**
- **Low fasting insulin**
- **High HDL**

And what causes these? Both triglycerides and fasting insulin are lower when sugar and processed carbs are eliminated or reduced. What raises HDL (the "good" cholesterol)? Surprise! It's eating saturated fat. So, in order to have the blood work of those who live to 100 or older, don't eat sugar or processed carbs, and do eat saturated fat.

For a more thorough analysis, read *The Great Cholesterol Myth Why Lowering Your Cholesterol Won't Prevent Heart Disease – And The Statin-Free Plan That Will,* by Johnny Bowden, Ph.D., C.N.S., and Steven Sinatra, M.D., F.A.C.C. [33]

Nurses' Health Study

The Nurses' Health Study is one of the longest-running studies of diet and disease. It was conducted by Harvard University. It studied 120,000 females beginning in the mid-1970's. It focused on the risk factors for cancer and heart disease. It included an exhaustive analysis of 84,129 of these women. It was published in the New England Journal of Medicine.

82% of coronary events could be attributed to 5 factors:

- Don't smoke
- Drink alcohol in moderation
- Engage in moderate to vigorous exercise for at least 30 minutes a day
- Maintain a healthy weight (BMI under 25)
- Eat a healthy, low glycemic index diet (low sugar and refined carbohydrates) with plenty of omega-3 fats and fiber

Note that lowering cholesterol is not on this list.
Avoiding fat is not on the list.

Statins

In any discussion about cholesterol, a word should be said about statins.

There are various forms of statins. In 2005, sales were estimated at 18.7 billion dollars in the United States. [57]   The best-selling statin is atorvastatin, more commonly known as Lipitor. In 2003, **Lipitor became the best-selling pharmaceutical in history. [58]**

Half of all men age 65-74 take a statin. Thirty-one percent of women over 75 take a statin. Wow! That's a lot of people.

Twenty-five percent of all Americans over the age of 45 are taking a statin.

Statins do seem to help middle-aged men with a history of heart problems. How much? The makers of Lipitor advertise a 33% reduction of heart attack risk.

Let's check this math.

But first let's talk about the difference between **relative risk reduction** and **absolute risk reduction**. **Absolute** risk reduction is the difference an intervention makes compared to a control group.   For example, out of 100 men, over 5 years, 3 of them would be expected to have a heart attack. Taking Lipitor reduces that number to 2 men out of 100. The absolute risk reduction is the difference between 3 heart attacks and 2 heart attacks, which is one.   One out of 100 is 1%. So, taking Lipitor reduces heart attacks by 1%. **The absolute risk reduction is 1%.**

Now let's look at the **relative risk reduction**. Relative risk is one number compared to another number, often expressed as a ratio or percentage. For example, if taking Lipitor reduces heart attacks from 3 to 2, what is the ratio or percentage reduction? Three minus two is one. Lipitor's effect is 1 fewer heart attacks out of 3 expected heart attacks. So, the **relative risk reduction is one out of three, or 33%.**

To summarize absolute risk reduction:

- Out of 100 men, over 5 years, 3 of them would be expected to have a heart attack.
- Taking Lipitor reduces that number from 3 to 2 men out of 100.
- The **absolute** risk reduction is 1% (one out of 100 fewer heart attacks)

Relative risk reduction:

- Out of 100 men, the heart attack rate went from 3 to 2.
- The reduction is one (3 minus 2) out of 3
- This is a 33% relative risk reduction.

The relative risk reduction is 33%, and that is the number that is advertised.

Lipitor reduces heart attacks by 33%. That sounds impressive, unless you look more carefully at the math.

"Relative risk is just another way to lie." [59]

Another study had similar numbers. For every 138 people treated for 5 years, one fewer dies. [57]

If you know that if you take Lipitor, your risk goes from 3 in 100 to 2 in 100 would you be willing to take it?

That probably depends.

What's the down side of taking a statin?

Side effects of the drug itself:

- The best-documented one is **muscle pain**, which occurs in 10-15% of patients.
- **Statins deplete your body of coenzyme Q10.** Low levels of Coenzyme Q10 are responsible for the muscle pain, weakness, and loss of energy. [33]
- **Statins can ruin your sex life.** Remember that cholesterol is

instrumental in making testosterone, estrogen, and progesterone.
- The brain depends on cholesterol to function well. It contains 25% of the body's cholesterol. **Statins may interfere with cognition and memory.**
- **Cholesterol is an essential part of every cell membrane.**
- Cholesterol helps make **vitamin D.**
- **Statins may deplete your brain of vitamin K2.** [60]
- **Statins can cause liver damage, nerve damage, short temper, cognitive decline, kidney failure, muscle damage, and if it is the heart muscle, it can cause death.** [61]

In addition:

- Statins have very little benefit for women, if any at all.
- Statins also have very little or no benefit for anyone over 47.

It does help middle-aged men with a history of heart attacks. That's it.

We are not told the truth about this best-selling drug in the history of pharmaceuticals.

I ask again, if you know all of this, would you take a statin?

Are women and men the same?

Most research on heart disease has been done on men. Only 20% of participants in clinical trials were women up to 1990, and only 25% after that. [62]

We have known as far back as the 1950's that women respond in a different way to fat and cholesterol. Women typically do not have heart attacks until after menopause which is 10-20 years after men begin having heart problems. [63]

The Framingham Study is one of the few studies that included women. It found that women over 50 showed no correlation between total cholesterol and heart attacks. And, since women under 50 rarely have heart issues, this means that **eating saturated fat is actually a good thing for women of all ages.**

Before menopause, they seem to be protected by estrogen, and after menopause, high total cholesterol is not an issue, at least up to total cholesterol levels of 294 mg/dl. [64] In **fact, women of any age have**

lower total mortality if they have high cholesterol.

This does not mean that they can eat anything. Just like men, if they eat sugars and processed flours, their triglycerides will go up, which is correlated with heart disease.

HDL is the best predictor of heart disease

The Framingham follow-up results showed, for men and women, age 40 to 90, HDL won the prize for the best predictor of risk of future heart disease. People with HDL levels below 35 mg/dl had eight times more heart attacks than people with an HDL level over 65 mg/dl. [65]

Blood work numbers can be rather easily changed. On a low-fat diet, you can expect the following:

· lower LDL cholesterol (the "bad" cholesterol)

This is considered a good outcome, BUT it also does the following:

- lower HDL cholesterol (the good cholesterol)
- triglycerides go up (high triglycerides are bad)

Why, then, do we target the lowering of LDL in medicine? Could it be that there is a drug that can lower LDL? Yes, it is the biggest drug money-maker of all time, statins. There evidently is no drug to easily raise HDL, so pharmaceutical companies prefer to ignore this very useful predictor in favor of something they can change with a drug. [39]

What raises HDL cholesterol? Eating saturated fat. There is no money in this for the drug companies.

Back to women:

Women have a more extreme reaction to the low-fat diet than men do, but not in a good way. For one year, Boeing employees followed a low-fat diet. [66] They found that:

· Total LDL dropped for both men and women, but not as much for women (a drop in LDL is supposed to be good, so not as helpful for women)

· HDL dropped one third more in women than in men (a drop in HDL increases heart attack risk, so much worse for women)

· Triglycerides rise more (high triglycerides increase heart attack risk, so worse for women)

In conclusion, a low-fat diet is not good for women's heart health.

What foods are high in cholesterol?

- Meats
- Whole milk
- Fresh egg yolks
- Butter and cheese
- Organ meats (liver, kidney, heart, tongue, tripe, pancreas, and giblets)
- Caviar (fish eggs)
- Cod liver oil
- Cold-water fish and shellfish (salmon, sardines, herring, mackerel, and shrimp)
- Lard
- Brains of animals [44]

Actually, only 15% of the body's cholesterol comes from our food. The other 85% is produced by our bodies, as needed. [53]

However, cholesterol-lowering drugs interfere with the body's ability to produce needed cholesterol. Other than the problems already mentioned, what do we notice about people with low cholesterol? Aggressive behavior and low self-control.

Controlling your cholesterol numbers with diet

I think we owe a huge debt to Dave Feldman. He is not a doctor. He is a software engineer. On his own he figured out many of the mysteries of cholesterol. This is what he did:

He started eating a ketogenic diet (high fat, low carbs) in 2015. He felt great. He went in for blood tests some months later and discovered that his cholesterol was 329. He is what is called a "hyper-responder", meaning that his cholesterol goes up much higher than most people when on a high fat, low carb (HFLC) diet.

He decided to take the test again two weeks later, but this time he ate less saturated fat. He lowered his total fat (3-day average) from 224 grams to 83 grams. What did he find on his blood tests? His total cholesterol went up. Strange. It went up almost 100 points, from 329 to 424. Wow! So, eating saturated fat was not what was causing his high cholesterol numbers.

He wanted to understand how cholesterol works, so he started getting lab tests every few days. He got 51 blood tests in the first 15 months of his project. [67]

Five years later, he had gathered an amazing amount of data on how to control cholesterol numbers.

What do I mean by cholesterol numbers? Primarily, I am talking about LDL, triglycerides, and HDL. These are some of the things your doctor checks with blood work. If you have high LDL numbers, your doctor will probably suggest you take a statin drug to bring down your LDL.

If you are eating a high fat, low carb diet (HFLC), you will probably have high HDL (good), low triglycerides (good), but also high LDL (considered bad by the medical community). But is LDL really bad for us? Let's look at what Dave Feldman found.

Keep in mind that he is doing what is called an **"N of one". That means that there is only one person in this study**. However, he has been talking about this on the internet, and posting for years, so may other people have joined him in testing their cholesterol.

Statistically, an "N of one" can be a very powerful study. If you can hold most things the same, such as the time of day you eat, and amount of exercise you do, and only change one thing, such as diet, and then measure an outcome (LDL numbers) that is considered a very powerful design for a study. If you can control the outcome (LDL numbers going up and down) by changing the one variable (diet, as in low fat or high fat), this shows causation not just correlation. If you can do this same thing with other people, even a few, that makes the results even more powerful.

What did he find?

White bread experiment

He normally eats a low carbohydrate diet. On this diet, he has low triglycerides and high HDL (both good) but high LDL (considered bad). What happens if he reverses this and eats highly processed carbohydrates and lean protein (high carb, low fat)?

He ate white bread (wonder bread) and processed lean meat turkey (protein with low fat) for a week and checked his numbers every day. What happened? Day by day, over 7 days, his LDL dropped from 296 (very high) to 83 (very low). Most doctors would be very pleased to see this. However, what happened to his other tests?

His triglycerides went from 78 (good) to 221 (very bad).

His glucose went from a high of 105 (good) to 177 (very bad).

His HDL went from 55 (acceptable) to 38 (bad). [68]

In other words, as he ate white bread and processed meat, his LDL dropped dramatically (most doctors would be happy), but his other measurements became dangerously unhealthy.

He offers $1000 to anyone who can produce a population that has high LDL, low triglycerides, and high HLD, as he usually does, and has cardiovascular problems. No takers yet.

In general, what has he found?

- **All cholesterol markers are highly influenced by the diet of just the previous three days.** We get blood tests, maybe once a year, and our medication decisions for the next year are made based on numbers that can fluctuate radically day by day.
- **All particle markers (LDL-P, which is the number of total LDL "boats") are highly influenced by the diet of just the previous five days.** Again, in only five days, these numbers can change dramatically.

Dave Feldman says that the **primary job of LDL is to distribute energy from fat.** We will die if our cells do not have energy available every minute of every day. **We have one hundred trillion cells that need to be fed.**

Where does this energy come from? After we eat, our bodies make triglycerides, load them into LDL "boats", and take them, through our blood stream, all over our bodies. About two thirds of these triglycerides go to the local fat (adipose tissue or subcutaneous fat), and about one third go directly to the cells. After we have used up the readily available triglycerides from food (typically abut 8 hours after eating), our bodies turn to the fat that is stored all over our bodies. It is a miraculous system that makes sure all of our cells are well fed. [67]

Why do some people accumulate so much fat? Partly this is because, in our culture, we are rarely in a "fasted state". If fasting happens about 8 hours after eating, and we are frequently eating all of our waking hours, when are we fasting? We never get there. If the cells are being continuously fed by triglycerides, after a while, the cells start refusing to accept any more triglycerides. The triglycerides get backed up in the blood system. This leads to high readings of triglycerides. These tend to be the small LDL particles. This is an unhealthy system. The small particles are the ones that damage the artery walls.

It is recommended that we wait at least 12 hours between our last meal of the day, and our first meal the next day to give our bodies a chance to be in the "fasted state" for some hours. Sixteen hours may be even better. This gives our bodies a chance to use up all of the available triglycerides in the blood, and begin using the energy stored in our fat cells.

Let's look at a healthy reason to have high LDL. What if we are lean and very athletic? We would need large amounts of triglycerides from our LDL "boats" in our blood. We couldn't count on much help from the stored fat in our bodies because there isn't much. Also, we would be using up the triglycerides as fast as they arrive in these LDL "boats" in our bloodstream. In this situation, our bodies will send more LDL "boats" full of triglycerides to feed the cells. These tend to be the large, "fluffy" LDL "boats". These do not damage our artery walls. This is a very healthy system.

Interestingly, in both cases, our LDL count will be high, but for different reasons, one healthy and one unhealthy.

How do we know which group we are in if our LDL count is high in both groups?

- We can measure whether or not the LDL particles are small or large. Small is bad and large is good.
- In the first group, triglycerides will be high in the blood. In the second group, triglycerides will be low because they are being used up as fast as they arrive. High triglycerides in the blood is bad.
- In the first group HDL will be low, and in the second group it will be high (high is good). [67]

How does cholesterol fit into this? Cholesterol is a passenger on the LDL "boat" along with the triglycerides, but it only gets off if it is needed for repair. If all is well, it travels back to the liver where it helps make hormones, etc., or it is sent on another LDL "boat" into the bloodstream to be there in case it is needed somewhere for repair.

How does insulin fit into this? The pancreas makes insulin. The job of insulin is to help energy go into the cells. If we are in a state of being continuously fed, our pancreas is constantly pumping insulin. When the cells start to refuse the energy, it is called "insulin insensitivity" or "insulin resistance". Eventually, if it is bad enough, the pancreas stops making insulin. This is called diabetes.

How does glucose fit into this? Carbohydrates become glucose. Excess protein can become glucose. They travel to the cells through the bloodstream, just like triglycerides do. They are another form of energy. There are so many ways for our cells to get energy because it is such a vital requirement. Again, without a constant energy supply, we die. However, note that the constant energy should not be from eating frequently. Some part of every day, we should be using up our stored fat.

In summary, a low carbohydrate, high fat diet, even high in saturated fats, will probably do these things to your blood work numbers:

- High HDL (good) -- the most important measurement in predicting future heart problems
- Low triglycerides – (good) a measure of eating fewer carbohydrates
- High LDL – only a problem if these are the small LDL's
- These numbers can change dramatically within 3-5 days with a change in diet

Dave Feldman did many experiments, dramatically changing his cholesterol numbers within just a few days. If you want to control your cholesterol numbers with food, check out his YouTube videos.

Keeping in mind that the primary job of LDL is to distribute energy from fat to all the cells of our body, is it really a good idea to interfere with this miraculous system by artificially lowering the liver's ability to make LDL "boats" by taking a statin drug? Something to consider if your doctor suggests you take a statin.

Macronutrient #2: Carbohydrates

The simplest way to look at all these associations, between obesity, heart disease, type 2 diabetes, metabolic syndrome, cancer, and Alzheimer's (not to mention the other conditions that also associate with obesity and diabetes, such as gout, asthma, and fatty liver disease), is that what makes us fat – the quality and quantity of carbohydrates we consume – also makes us sick.

--Gary Taubes [69]

Carbohydrates are fruits and vegetables (healthy), but also sugar and flour (unhealthy).

Eat an unlimited amount of non-starchy vegetables.

This should be most of what you eat every day. Some researchers say up to 80% of our diets should be fruits and vegetables (by volume). Go for many different colors. Different colors have different micronutrients. For example, orange vegetables, such as carrots, have beta carotene.

Non-starchy vegetables are also low in calories and sugars, so eat unlimited amounts of non-starchy vegetables.

Starchy vegetables, like white potatoes, are considered by some nutritionists to be not as healthy as non-starchy vegetables. They have a higher glycemic index, so they can spike blood sugar, just like white flour and sugar. However, even though they are higher in calories than non-starchy vegetables, and have a higher glycemic index, they are very filling and are a "real food". Also, they are relatively low in calories.

The choice of whether to eat starchy vegetables and bread is where many researchers disagree. Some say to eat beans, whole grains, and potatoes (Esselstein). Others say to minimize these and eat a diet high in healthy fats (Mercola, Hyman).

More important than the glycemic index is the glycemic load of the meal. All of the things eaten together add up to the glycemic load. If you eat half of a potato along with a variety of other vegetables, this leads to a lower glycemic load in the meal, compared to eating just the potato. A lower glycemic load keeps blood sugar from spiking.

Some vegetables are healthier than others.

Non-starchy vegetables -- healthiest to eat

- Kale, Onions, Garlic, Lemon, Spinach, Cabbage, Bell pepper, Broccoli, Cucumber, Cauliflower, Asparagus, Eggplant, Zucchi, Ginger, Greens (a good variety), Celery, Green beans, Fennel, Leeks, Mushrooms, Brussel sprouts, Collard greens, Tomatoes, Watercress, Oregano, Cilantro, Parsley, Basil, Thyme, Rosemary, and sage.
- All vegetable sprouts, such as broccoli, mustard, and kale.
- Seeds (all seeds and nuts), such as almonds, chia, hemp, and pumpkin, although there is quite a range.
- Berries (all berries), such as blueberries and strawberries

Starchy vegetables -- eat in limited amounts or not at all

This is a list of common starchy vegetables. The serving sizes (½ cup to 1 cup), have about 15 grams of carbohydrate, 3 grams of protein and 80 calories. [70]

- White Potatoes (1/2 cup mashed, 1/2 cup roasted or 10 to 15 French fries)
- Yams (1/2 cup)
- Corn -- really a grain (1/2 cup)
- Green Peas (1/2 cup)
- Parsnips (1/2 cup)
- Sweet Potatoes (1/2 cup)
- Winter Squash, such as acorn or butternut squash (~3/4 cup)
- Beets (1 cup)
- Carrots (1 cup)

Fruit

Get a good variety of fruit to get a range of micronutrients, but fruit is full of sugar and calories, so not so much in quantity. **So, large variety but small amounts.**

Fruit has natural sugar, and it's better for you than cane sugar or high fructose corn syrup, but it is still sugar. A huge plus of eating whole fruit rather than fruit juice is that fruit comes with fiber. The fiber slows down the digestion so that the blood sugar doesn't spike as much. In addition, some fruit has low sugar, such as blueberries, and some fruit has a high sugar content, such as grapes. See section on sugar.

Beans

Beans are great for protein and fiber. Around the world, many of the population groups that are known for their longevity [1] have one thing in common: they eat beans.

However, there are other authors who say to never eat beans because of the high carbohydrates. (79)

Grains

Grains have a high glycemic index, and may spike blood sugar.

Many researchers say that all grains should be avoided because of this. See chapter on wheat.

Are starchy carbohydrates healthy?

The Tukisenta in Papua New Guinea were studied between 1966-68. [11] Sweet potatoes were 90% of their calories -- 1000 different kinds of sweet potatoes. They occasionally ate pork and chicken. Their diet consisted of:

- 94.6% carbs
- 3% protein
- 2.4% fat

How is their health? They were lean and fit and healthy with:

- No obesity
- No diabetes
- No or rare heart disease
- No macular degeneration

In addition, in many of the Bues Zones, the indiginous diets were primarily starchy plants. The people had very few diseases and impressive longevity. See chapter on Blue Zones.

If carbohydrates drive insulin and insulin drives fat, how can we explain this? Maybe it is refined carbohydrates (sugar and flour) that are the problem, not so much whole plant foods.

(Personal note:)

Honestly, I don't have a good answer for this. Some people thrive on whole plant foods, including starchy carbs.

I avoid all starchy carbohydrates because I have noticed that my balance is worse, not only from sugar, flour and alcohol, but also if I eat a potato or too much sweet fruit.

Summary of carbohydrates

Eating a large variety of fruits and vegetables provides the nutrition that our cells need, and helps keep our gut bacteria healthy. Eat mostly non-starchy vegetables. Eat some fruit, but not too much because of the high sugar content. Avoid processed carbohydrates such as wheat flour.

(Personal Note:)

Here is a **list of the fresh fruits and vegetables that I eat over the course of a year.** I don't like all vegetables, but I like to try new foods, so I tend to eat almost anything at least once. I highlighted the ones I have almost every week.

Broccoli, cauliflower, Brussel sprouts, **tomatoes, green beans, onions, carrots, celery,** basil, sage, oregano, thyme, **cinnamon,** mint, marjoram, **fennel,** red, purple and white **cabbage,** (purple is my favorite), kale, **spinach,** leeks, **blueberries,** raspberries, strawberries, blackberries, chia seeds, hemp seeds, pumpkin seeds, **almonds, cashews,** sunflower seeds, walnuts, **pecans, pistachios,** oats, **mushrooms** (various kinds), beets, squash (various kinds), sweet potatoes, yams, parsnips, turnips, corn, white potatoes (fingerling are my favorites), radish (daikon is my favorite), zucchini, lettuce greens, **cilantro,** parsley, **lemons,** oranges, grapefruit, **bell peppers (red,** yellow, and orange), eggplant, **garlic,** ginger, **mustard, asparagus,** cucumber, grapes, raisins, pineapple, mango, **bananas, sprouts of all kinds (broccoli, kale, mustard, and radish are my favorites),** persimmons, and pomegranates.

How many do you eat? You might want to try some new vegetables. Your body will thank you.

Check out my YouTube videos on how to make healthy foods taste terrific. *(Creating Health with Dr. Andrea Covert)*

Macronutrient #3: Protein

It is generally recommended that we multiply our body weight by .34 and eat that many grams of protein per day. A woman of 120 pounds should eat 40 grams of protein per day. A man weighing 180 pounds should eat 60 grams of protein per day. Those who eat lots of meat and dairy may be eating too much protein, and those eating a vegan diet many not be eating enough protein, according to this formula. There are some people who should be eating more than this, such as athletes. They may need up to one gram per pound of body weight.

If we don't eat enough protein, we may lose muscle mass. If we eat too much protein, it is made into glucose and may spike blood sugar.

How much vegetable protein do we need to eat to get enough?

It is actually quite difficult to get 40-60 grams of protein a day without eating any animal products or soy, and without supplementing.

Some common proteins: [71]

Food	Protein (grams)
Animal sources	
3 ounces tuna, salmon, haddock, or trout	21
3 ounces cooked turkey or chicken	19
6 ounces plain Greek yogurt	17
½ cup cottage cheese	14
1 cup of milk	8
1 egg	6
Non-animal sources	
½ cup cooked beans	8
1 cup cooked pasta	8
¼ cup or 1 ounce of nuts (all types)	7
(Soy to be discussed later)	

In order to get the recommended 40 grams of protein for a 120-pound female, she would have to eat 2.5 cups of beans a day, or 5 cups of pasta per day. That is way too many calories. So, my conclusion is that we need to eat animal products to meet those protein requirements, or take supplements (such as protein powder) to get the recommended protein. Since these supplements are processed foods, which I try to avoid, that really only leaves eating animal products to get adequate protein.

But the question is: do we really need this level of protein?

Dr. Esselstyn [30] says that we get plenty of protein by just eating healthy fruits, vegetables and whole grains. He did a research study with 24 people who had advanced heart disease. Many of them had had bypass surgery and other forms of medical intervention, and were essentially "on death's door". He supervised them in eating a whole-food plant-based diet. No fats. No animal products. At the 20-year mark, 18 were still alive with no more cardiovascular issues. At the 27-year mark, 14 were still alive. Very impressive.

His son, Rip Esselstein, wrote a book called *The Engine 2 Diet.* [72] has been a vegan his whole life (or so I understand). He was a triathlete in his early years, then became a fireman. He promotes the vegan diet. He has written books and has made 2 movies. I highly recommend them. It evidently works well for him.

Another impressive example: Dr. Ruth Heinrich had stage 4 breast cancer in her early 40's. It had spread to many other parts of her body. She had surgery to remove a golf-ball sized lump in her breast. Instead of undergoing the recommended chemotherapy and radiation, she instead started eating a whole-food plant-based diet. Within 2 months her blood work numbers were in the normal range. At the two-year mark, she just had one small lump in her lung. She later changed her diet to a plant-based raw food diet. She is now in her 80's and is a triathlete. No cancer. People ask her what she does for protein. She says she gets plenty of protein from her raw fruits, vegetables and grains. So, she cured herself of cancer, became a triathlete, and does not show any symptoms of low protein intake. [73]

In addition, there is the Blue Zone of Okinawa, where the people live to 100 eating 97% plants. They must be getting adequate protein from vegetables to live to over 100 in good health.

I don't know what is correct with regard to how much protein we really need. However, I am going to accept that we need the .37 grams of protein per pound of body weight, for purposes of discussing what to eat.

So, if we accept that the amount of protein is fairly fixed, we have to choose our additional calories from fats or carbohydrates.

We have been told to eat low-fat (particularly saturated fats) for the last 50 years, so most people have chosen to get their calories from sugar, vegetable oils, and white flour.

This diet has led to an explosion of diseases.

(Personal Note)

There is so much contradictory evidence about how much protein to eat. From trying different amounts of protein in my diet,

I have concluded that the .34 grams of protein per pound of body weight works well for me at this point in my life. However, most of my adult life I ate the recommended low-fat diet, which included small amounts of meat. Consequently, I was not getting very much animal protein, and I seemed to do just fine.

I increased my protein because I was having trouble losing weight. I added more animal protein when I was about 64. I added more animal fat when I was 67. I feel much better. After adding the fat, I am not as hungry, I am no longer easily cold, and I have lost my cravings for sweets. As we age, I have read that we need more protein to maintain muscle mass, perhaps because our bodies don't process protein as efficiently.

You decide what is best for you.

Protein consists of different amino acids.

Nine proteins are called "essential amino acids" because the human body cannot synthesize them from other compounds at the level needed for normal growth, so they must be obtained from food. Some foods, like animal products, have all nine proteins, and in the correct balance. There are some vegetables and grains that have complete proteins, and there are many vegetables that have some or most of our essential amino acids.

We use amino acids to build healthy cells, synthesize enzymes and hormones, build antibodies, guard against infection and build muscle. It is also an important source of energy and helps us to feel full after a meal.

Too little or too much is harmful.

Not enough protein may lead to:

- trouble losing weight
- trouble gaining muscle mass
- poor concentration
- muscle, bone and joint pain
- low immunity
- slow wound healing
- diabetes
- moodiness and mood swings
- low energy levels and fatigue

- a sluggish metabolism

Too much protein:

Excess protein is turned into glucose. Too much glucose is one of the primary reasons we have so many health problems.

Complete Proteins

What foods contain complete proteins, meaning they have all of the amino acids we need?

Animal proteins contain all of the amino acids we need in the right ratio.

There are also some vegetables and grains that have complete proteins, such as quinoa and soy. In addition, there are some protein combinations that make a complete protein, like beans and rice.

Animal Proteins

Meat is an excellent source of protein. However, eating meat is a hotly debated subject by the experts in food research (see section on meat). Some recommend unlimited amounts of meat. Others recommend no meat ever. That's quite a range. It is very unclear in the research. Short term, there seems to be no problem with eating limited amounts of meat. I know there are many reasons vegetarians and vegans avoid meet for ethical reasons. I am not covering these here in any detail. I am just focusing on the health benefits. However, there is a huge difference between conventionally raised animals and grass-fed animals both in terms of kindness to the animals and our health.

Reasons to eliminate all conventionally grown animal products (animals that are taken off the range, to the feed lots, to fatten up for the last few months of their lives):

- We feed our livestock many kinds of foods that they are not genetically programmed to eat. Let's look at beef. **Cattle are meant to eat wild grasses.** They are raised on wild grasses, but then they are moved to feed lots to fatten up. There we feed them corn and soy, typically grown with herbicides and pesticides (poisons). Corn makes them fatter (corn-fed beef). They don't eat corn normally. **Corn is very high in omega 6's, so we are getting abnormally high amounts if omega 6's in our diet along**

with the poison.

- **Conditions are very harsh** on the feed lots.
- They are also given **antibiotics,** both for infection, because they are all packed together in unhealthy conditions, and because the antibiotics help them grow faster. The faster the animals grow, the lower the cost, so if antibiotics can make the animals grow faster, that saves the ranchers money. However, as antibiotics kill certain bacteria, that leaves the antibiotic-resistant bacteria to take over. Different and stronger antibiotics are needed to kill these bacteria. In this way, we are selecting for bacteria that antibiotics cannot kill. Partly because of this practice, antibiotics are losing their ability to cure humans of our diseases. There are now bacteria that no kind of antibiotics will kill. We use about 24 million pounds of antibiotics per year in America. Out of this, about 19 million pounds are used in animal feed. We need to stop doing this if we want antibiotics to continue to be effective in saving human lives.
- They are also fed **hormones.** Hormones make the cattle grow faster. Giving them hormones is possibly why American girls are maturing earlier and earlier.
- **Depletion of our aquifers** (underground sources of water) and global freshwater supplies, because 70% of the world's freshwater is used to grow animals for human consumption.
- They eat food with pesticides and herbicides, so there is a residual of poison in the meat. [46]

When we eat animals treated like this, we are bringing all of those unhealthy things into our bodies: omega 6's, poison, antibiotics and hormones. See section on omega 3's and 6's for a full explanation.

Eating pasture-fed meat (animals that live all of their lives on the range) avoids all of this. In addition, we get a healthy dose of vitamin K2 (see section on vitamin K2).

Reasons to eat grass-fed meats (animals that eat what they are supposed to eat, and are left on the pasture their entire lives):

- Grass-fed animals **don't need antibiotics** because they are not being fed foods that bloat their stomachs.
- There are **2-5 times more omega-3 fats in grass fed meat,** and lower levels of omega-6 fats. The ratio of omega-6 to omega-3 is about 1.5 to 1 in grass-fed meat, while grain-fed beef has about a

7.5 to 1 ratio (we are aiming for about a 1 to 1 ratio).

- Grass-fed meat has **more vitamins and anti-oxidants**. [46]

I recommend that you consider buying pasture-fed animal products, even though it does cost more. If you are concerned about the added cost, consider eating a smaller portion of meat and a larger portion of vegetables and healthy fats. Your body will thank you.

What if everyone knew that they were eating meat that is unhealthy and the only bought meat:

- **that was pasture-raised.**
- **free of hormones and antibiotics.**

Would food really cost more?

What are the true costs of eating meat that is moved to the feed lots to fatten up? Perhaps this practice is contributing to heart disease, cancer, diabetes, obesity, autoimmune diseases, pollution, etc. In addition, our antibiotics are now failing us.

Is it really cheaper to eat this way? The large corporations make more money, but we pay the rest of the bill.

Europe has been concerned about this for a long time. **In 1989, the European Union banned the importation of meat that contained artificial beef growth hormones.** These were estradiol, progesterone, testosterone, zeranol, melengestrol, acetate, and trenbolone acetate. All of these were licensed for use in the United States and Canada. Since then, there has been a legal battle over importing beef from the United States. The battle includes the labeling of meat products with hormones.

This battle with exporting our beef to Europe has awakened interest in the United States. In a study done in 2002, 85% of respondents wanted mandatory labeling on beef produced with growth hormones. (Lusk & Fox, 2002, April) Partly out of concern for this, organic meats and poultry is the fastest growing agricultural sector. From 2002-2003, it grew 77.8%, accounting for $23 billion in the entire organic food market. [74]

If you are going to eat meat, I suggest that you eat pasture-fed and "pasture-finished" animals that have not been given antibiotics or growth hormones.

Eat eggs from pasture-fed chickens (and for the vitamin K2).

Eat cheese and butter from pasture-fed cows (also for the K2).

In the recipe section, I do include eggs, cheese, and sour cream.

Humans are clearly meant to eat some meat and animal products. We need vitamins B12 and K2 (found in animal products and very difficult to get any other way). They can be taken as supplements, but I believe that we are meant to eat real food, so I have included real food to cover what I believe we need to eat in a day.

I have found that it is very hard to get the recommended amount of protein without eating meat or animal products and without eating soy.

In conclusion, if you want to eat meat, go ahead. It is safest to eat pasture-fed and pasture-finished meat. Eat animal products from pasture-fed animals. No antibiotics. No growth hormones. Whether it is best to make it a small part of your diet or a large part is still unclear. You decide.

Eggs

Eggs are an excellent source of animal protein. There are 6 grams of protein per egg. In addition, pasture-fed chicken eggs have vitamin K2. The yolks also contain some vitamin D.

What to look for in eggs:

Pasture raised, organic, no antibiotics, no hormones.

Eggs from hens fed in pastures have been found to have:

- ⅔ more vitamin A
- 2 times more omega 3 fatty acids
- 3 times more Vitamin E
- 7 times more beta carotene
- 50% more folic acid
- 70% more vitamin B12
- 4-6 times more vitamin D than conventional eggs
- They are an excellent source of Vitamin K2.[138]
- ⅓ less cholesterol
- ¼ less saturated fat

Eating 2 pasture-raised eggs probably supplies all of the vitamin K2 needed for the day. I say "probably" because research on K2 is rather new. [31]

What is pasture-fed, free-range, cage free, etc.? The names can be very confusing and misleading.

Pasture-fed. This is the one to buy. The chickens should have enough acreage to roam in the sunshine and eat what is in the field. They may eat worms, bugs, seeds, etc. The shells should not be all the same color, and the yolk should have a variation in color, but all the yolks should be a bright yellow, orange, or even red/orange. The variation in color is due to the fact that they are not all eating the same thing. The bright orange yolk is from eating things in the field that have beta-carotene. In addition, these chickens and eggs have K2, a vital nutrient, that they get from eating real food in the sunshine. Sometimes these chickens are given supplemental food. Check to make sure that they are not being given chicken feed that contains corn, soy or wheat.

Free range. These chickens get some time outdoors. This is good for the chickens, but not better for us. They are probably fed GMO corn and soy. They probably have added hormones and antibiotics. Yolks are pale yellow.

Cage free. This means that they are not kept in tiny cages. They are still probably indoors, but they mingle with each other. They are probably fed GMO corn and soy, and receive antibiotics and hormones. The yolks are pale yellow.

Conventionally raised. These sad chickens are kept in a small cage, fed GMO corn and soy, and given antibiotics and hormones. Some companies cut off their beaks to keep them from pecking each other. These are sad miserable little chickens. All of the other variations are better for the chickens. Yolks are pale yellow.

Note: Because chickens are fed GMO corn and soy, the chickens and the eggs probably have a residue of glyphosate in them, so you are getting a steady flow of poison if you eat these foods. The glyphosate doesn't kill "you", but they kill the bacteria in your gut. A healthy gut microbiome is essential for your overall health. Also, the chickens and eggs can only supply you with the micronutrients that they eat. The pasture-fed chickens have a huge range of micronutrients available to them. All of the others have a very limited range of micronutrients to eat.

What to look for in cheese and milk products:

I recommend only eating milk products from pasture-fed cows. This has natural K2, and should have no antibiotics or hormones, and no poisons.

Gouda from pasture fed cows has the additional advantage of having more Vitamin K2 content from the bacteria that make this kind of cheese. Brie cheese has less K2, but is still a good source. The bacteria that make gouda and brie add to the K2 in the cheese. There are 7 grams of protein in one ounce of cheese.

Greek yogurt has the additional advantage of providing good probiotics. It typically has 23 grams of protein per cup.

Consider drinking raw milk from pasture-fed cows. "Raw milk" means that it comes to you just as the cow made it. It is not pasteurized (heated to kill bacteria) or homogenized (a process that keeps the cream from floating to the top of the milk). Homogenized and pasteurized milk is somewhat damaged in terms of health value. However, you need to be very confident that the source of the raw milk is reliable. If the milk is unpasteurized, the cows need to be really healthy.

Try to buy milk that has type A2 casein (see chapter on what your ancestors ate).

Vegetable sources of complete protein

Do we need to eat complete proteins with every bite? Probably not, but there are varying opinions about this. I think it is safest to supply our bodies, as much as possible, with complete proteins. The good news is that there are many vegetables and grains that can supply our amino acid needs.

1. Quinoa
Full of fiber, iron, magnesium, and manganese. Quinoa is a complete protein. It is an excellent substitute for rice. It is actually a seed, not a grain. However, it is a starchy seed, so it may spike blood sugar. Quinoa has a glycemic index of 53.

2. Buckwheat
Buckwheat is not a type of wheat. It's a fruit seed, and a relative of rhubarb. It has no gluten and makes a good substitute for wheat. It is also not a grain. Buckwheat has a glycemic index of 45-51.

3. Soy
I avoid soy because it is almost exclusively a GMO food. Also, it is

very high in omega-6 fatty acids. I try to eat only "real food". Other than edamame, most soy is processed, so I avoid it.

However, I realize that for vegans, this may be their only real choice if they want to get enough protein without eating animal products.

Soy is a complete protein. If you choose to use soy as a protein source, I recommend organic edamame.

4. Rice and Beans

One of the best sources of non-animal protein is also one of the easiest and cheapest. Most beans are low in methionine and high in lysine, while rice is low in lysine and high in methionine. Combined, they make a complete protein.

5. Hummus and Whole Wheat Pita

The protein in wheat is deficient only in lysine. But chickpeas, like other beans, have plenty of lysine, so here again you have an excellent complete protein when they are combined. See the chapter on wheat before making this your favorite protein food.

6. Peanut Butter

Peanuts are a complete source of protein. They are not really a nut, but a bean.

7. Hemp seed

Hemp seeds contain significant amounts of all nine essential amino acids (though it's too low in lysine to be considered complete), as well as plenty of magnesium, zinc, iron, and calcium. They also have omega-3s. Their omega-3 to omega-6 ratio is about 1 to 4. That is still in the acceptable range.

8. Chia Seeds

An excellent source of protein, omega-3 fatty acids, fiber, iron, magnesium, manganese, phosphorus, calcium, zinc, and antioxidants. [75]

9. Nuts and seeds

All nuts and seeds are a good source of protein, but they are not a complete protein. Almonds win the prize for the most nutrition.

When the diets of the Seventh Day Adventists (one of the groups that lives the longest) were analyzed, they found that those who ate nuts and seeds lived up to 7 years longer than the others. That is a good recommendation for adding nuts and seeds to our diets.

Note: I am not recommending grains, beans, rice, or soy (other than edamame), but for those who are choosing a low-fat diet, or avoiding animal products, these are some alternatives.

Also of note: Vegetable proteins have the additional advantage of adding fiber (meat has no fiber) and providing essential nutrients.

One big plus of eating animal sources of protein is that animal products provide vitamin B12 and K2. However, nattto (a fermented soybean product) has vitamin K2. This is a very popular source of K2 in Japan, and may be good for vegans to consider. In addition, fish have a very usable source of omega 3 fatty acid. It is harder for our bodies to use vegetable sources.

Fish

Sadly, most or all fish may be contaminated with mercury and other human-caused contaminants. In choosing which fish to eat, look for fish at the bottom of the food chain that are not very old when eaten.

Fish like shark, at the top of the food chain, that live long lives, are a poor choice. Because they live long lives, they spend many years eating smaller fish. Every time they eat another fish, the mercury and other poisons from the smaller fish accumulate in the shark.

We want to eat the fish near the bottom of the food chain that also live a short life. What is that?

Wild Alaskan sockeye salmon wins!

Question: But aren't we overfishing? Isn't it better for the environment to buy farmed salmon?

Answer: Wild Alaskan salmon fishing is carefully controlled. They let enough salmon lay their eggs to produce the next generation, then the rest can be caught. There are some years that 20,000 salmon are in the rivers, but only 2,000 are needed to produce enough eggs.

Salmon is not only an excellent source of protein, but also contains one of the best sources of omega 3 fatty acid.

It is only 3-4 years old when it swims upstream to reproduce. Sockeye salmon primarily eat zooplankton. They also eat small aquatic organisms such as shrimp. Juveniles also eat insects. Because of their diet, they do not accumulate so much mercury. Some other species of salmon eat small crustaceans like shrimps or small fish. Still good, but not as good as wild sockeye.

The Monterey Bay Aquarium has a program called Seafood Watch which ranks fish on the basis of (1) contaminants (2) Omega 3 content and (3) sustainability.

The Monterey Bay Aquarium gives a high rating to these fish:

- Atlantic mackerel from Canada and the U.S.
- Wild caught Pacific sardines
- Wild caught salmon from Alaska
- Wild caught canned salmon from Alaska

Fish to avoid:

- **Bluefin Tuna.** They have high levels of mercury and PCB's. Their populations have been overfished.
- **Orange Roughy.** This fish lives 100 years or more. Therefore, it has a very high concentration of mercury.
- **Salmon (Atlantic, farmed in pens).** These fish are tightly packed together and often have parasites and diseases. They are given antibiotics, bringing up the same problem we have with beef. They are often fed corn, raising their omega 6 content.
- **Halibut (Atlantic, wild).** These fish can live 50 years, so they tend to have high a mercury content. They have also been overfished.

Then there are the recommended "smash" fish:

- Salmon
- Mackerel
- Anchovies
- Sardines
- Herring

These are all great sources of omega 3's and vitamin D, are low in mercury, and are all sustainable.

The fish dilemma:

Just as mercury and other contaminants accumulate in fish, these same poisons accumulate in us over a lifetime. Therefore, it is a difficult decision.

Should you eat fish for its excellent omega 3 content, or should you avoid fish because of the accumulation of contaminants? Tough decision.

Personal Note

The only fish I eat is wild Alaskan Sockeye salmon. I eat it about once a week. I buy it frozen from Costco.

Summary of proteins:

This is a tough subject because by eating just fruits and vegetables (excluding soy) it is hard to get the recommended amount of protein in a day. The US Department of Agriculture recommends that we eat at least .34 grams of protein per pound of body weight. A woman of 120 points should get about 40 grams of protein per day. A man of 180 pounds should get about 60 grams of protein.

To get this amount, we need to add either meat (or other animal products) or soy. On the other hand, Dr. Esselstyn [30] says we get plenty of protein from vegetables, and that we should not worry about the recommended daily amount. In addition, some Blue Zones thrive on almost exclusively vegetables.

Take Away

Fats

- Eat healthy fats, not unhealthy fats, from 0 to 80% of calories (depending on the research, see what works for you).

Carbohydrates

- Eat an unlimited amount of non-starchy organic vegetables (80% of volume).
- Eat a variety of fruits, but limited quantity due to the sugar content.
- Limit or eliminate whole grains, pasta, whole-grain bread, beans, potatoes, and other starchy vegetables if you are eating a high-fat, low-carb diet. If you are eating a low-fat, high carb diet, these things may be fine. Even on a low-carb diet, you may want to sometimes have a high-carb day with starchy vegetables (such as beans and potatoes).

Proteins

- Aim for one third of your body weight in grams of protein (120-pound woman eats 40 grams of protein)
- Eat grass-fed meat and pasture-fed chickens and eggs, and organic pork.
- Eat wild-caught Alaskan salmon or other healthy fish once a week.
- Or for vegans or vegetarians, eat vegetable combinations that make complete proteins, or soy (which contains all essential amino acids).

In all groups, do not eat processed or packaged foods that contain sugar, wheat flour, or vegetable oils.

Chapter 4

The Big Killers

Sugar -- Enemy #1?

"Sugar was once called "white death". It deserves 100% of this title."
                    --Natasha Campbell-McBride

One third of all adults are obese, two-thirds are overweight, and almost one in seven is diabetic . . . one in four to five will die of cancer, "yet the prime suspects for the dietary trigger of these conditions have been, until the last decade, treated as little worse than a source of harmless pleasure"
                    --Gary Taubes, [76]

Gary Taubes wrote *The Case Against Sugar*, [76] published in 2016, detailing why he believes sugar is the driving force behind all, or most, of our chronic diseases. He includes sucrose and high fructose corn syrup in his definition of "sugar".

Sugar (and wheat flour and seed oils, to be discussed later) are the main reasons people have chronic illnesses.

In 2008 the average intake of sugar in the US was 76.7 grams per day, which equals 19 teaspoons or 306 calories.

Excess sugar consumption has been associated with obesity, type II diabetes, cardiovascular disease, certain cancers, tooth decay, non-alcoholic fatty liver disease, and many other illnesses.

Sugar is in almost all processed foods. **What does it do that is so damaging?**

- It **overloads the body with glucose.**
- This causes the **blood sugar to spike, then crash.**
- This creates **damage to the lining of the blood vessels.**
- It leaves us **hungry and tired** and craving more sugar.
- It is **bad for our gut bacteria** by crowding out healthy gut bacteria and feeding unhealthy bacteria.
- It **damages our immune system**, in part by feeding unhealthy gut bacteria.
- It **uses up the vitamins and minerals** that are needed to process the sugar, leaving a shortage of these vital elements, so that they cannot do the rest of their job (see section on magnesium)
- We tend to **eat too much,** so we gain weight.
- If we are eating sugar, we are not hungry for healthy vegetables and healthy fats, the food we should be eating.

To minimize sugars in the diet, avoid these foods:

- Soft drinks
- Fruit juices
- Candies and sweets
- Baked goods
- Fruits canned in syrup
- Low-Fat or Diet Foods
- Dried fruits
- All processed foods
- All added sugars

Natural sugars are fine to eat, such as fruit, but even some fruits have a high sugar content. The good news about fruit is that it contains fiber, so the glycemic index is lower when eaten as a whole fruit.

I recommend that people eat a good variety of fruits, but not too much because of the possible spike in blood sugar, and minimize the fruits that are especially high in sugar, such as grapes and pineapple.

Sources of sugar in real food

Fat has no sugar.

Protein has no sugar, but if you eat too much protein, your body will make glucose (bad), so stick to the .34 grams of protein per pound of body weight per day. Athletes may need more.

Carbohydrates. That is where the sugar is.

All non-starchy vegetables are great. Eat lots of these. They tend to be very low in sugar.

Starchy vegetables and grains (white potatoes, rice, pasta, bread, flour, etc.). Eat limited amounts of these, or none at all. These can spike blood sugar as much or more than table sugar.

Fruit. Most fruit is good to eat in small amounts, but eat a large variety to get a good range of micronutrients. However, some varieties of fruit have such a high sugar content that they should be treated like a dessert (to be eaten in small amounts occasionally).

These fruits are high in sugars:

- Grapes
- Pears
- Watermelon
- Cherries
- Mangoes

These fruits are low in sugars:

- Lemons and limes
- Raspberries
- Strawberries
- Blackberries
- Kiwis
- Grapefruit
- Avocado
- Cantaloupe
- Oranges
- Peaches

All sugar is still sugar. Bad. But let's face it, most of us like sweet things.

If you must use a sweetener, use one of these. However, keep in mind that eating anything sweet may trigger cravings for sweets that could last for days. *My comments are in italics.*

- Banana. *My favorite sweetener.*
- Raw honey from organic farms. *I use this, but sparingly. For me,*

it does trigger cravings.
- Molasses.
- Maple syrup. (Organic)
- Dates.
- Agave nectar has been considered a "healthy alternative" to sugar, because of its slightly lower glycemic index (good), but it has a high fructose content (bad). It is also quite processed. It has sweetness with very little additional flavor. I recommend avoiding this.
- Stevia is a plant with leaves that taste sweet. Using these leaves as a sweetener is just eating real food (good). However, any other form of stevia is not a real food. I recommend avoiding it. Even artificial sweeteners can trigger cravings.

Do not eat:

- All artificial sweeteners
- White sugar
- Brown sugar
- High fructose corn syrup (HFCS)
- Hydrated cane juice
- Syrup
- Brown rice syrup
- Cane sugar
- Sugars with the suffix "ose" (sucrose, fructose, glucose, lactose, maltose, dextrose, etc.)
- Any packaged foods that have sugars (breakfast cereals, bread, ketchup, salad dressing, sweetened yogurt, granola, barbecue sauce, pickles, coffee with creamers or sugar, sweet tea, smoothies, many mixed drinks, sweet wines, peanut butter with sugar, etc.)

Fructose

Fructose is especially damaging. Why is this? **Fructose can only be metabolized by the liver.** Eating fructose is one reason we have such an increase in non-alcoholic fatty liver disease. Having a fatty liver is the source of many other diseases. Let's review some basics about sucrose, fructose and glucose.

Starches (like potatoes) are broken down into **glucose** molecules and are absorbed by the intestines. The glycemic index measures how much blood sugar rises when a certain food is eaten. "Glucose is the primary sugar found in the blood . . . Every cell in the body can use glucose, and it circulates freely throughout the body. . . Certain cells, such as red blood cells, can *only* use glucose for energy." [77]

Table sugar (sucrose) is half glucose and half fructose. High fructose corn syrup is 55% fructose and 45% glucose. Pure fructose is rarely consumed, except as an ingredient in some processed foods. [77]

Fructose, interestingly, initially looked like it might be a healthier source of sweetener because it does not raise blood sugar. It also does not raise insulin levels. Sounds healthier? Not really. Why?

Every cell in the body can use glucose for energy. Eighty percent of the glucose is metabolized and used by cells all over the body. Only 20% is left for the liver to metabolize.

By contrast, **none of the cells in our bodies can metabolize fructose. Only the liver can metabolize fructose.**

The liver makes fructose into glucose, lactose, and glycogen. Consequently, if a steady large amount of fructose is eaten, the liver becomes overwhelmed by the amount of fructose it has to deal with. This creates fatty liver disease. [77]

How long have we known that sugar is deadly?

John Yudkin wrote a book called *Pure, White and Deadly How Sugar Is Killing Us and What We Can Do to Stop It* [78] in 1972 (first called *Sweet and Dangerous*).

In this book he talks about how the world sugar production increased from .25 tons in 1800 to 70 tons in 1970, to 101 tons in 1982. He goes on to say that the U.S. per capita consumption of **soft drinks went from 40 in 1950 to 300 in 1980.**

He associates sugar consumption with many diseases, and suggests that perhaps sugar should be banned.

He equates the lack of understanding about sugar with what the tobacco industry did to prevent the truth coming out with regard to smoking. He says that "freedom of choice exists only if there is freedom of information. The sugar industry has constantly attempted to prevent the public from being informed about the harmful effects of sugar."

Yudkin ends his book by saying, "It is difficult to avoid the conclusion that this is the result of the vigorous, continuing, and expanding activities of the sugar interests." [78]

So, interestingly, in 1972, we knew that the scientific literature

supported that sugar was "deadly", and yet, we continue to treat sugar as a harmless indulgence.

Interesting sugar story

I saw a friend drink a Starbucks Caffe Mocha the other day. He drank the whole thing. It was the 40 oz size. I looked at the sugar content: 105 grams of sugar. I asked him if he realized this. He did not. It said 21 grams per serving. He thought it was 21 grams total, but there were 5 servings per bottle.

This is the equivalent of five 8-oz cokes. You probably wouldn't have five cokes for breakfast.

Personal Note

I made the decision to not eat any added sugar. Once I got used to it, I found that food tastes delicious without the sugar. Our tastes adjust. In addition, I lost my strong cravings for sweets. Making the decision was much harder than actually doing it. I recommend going "cold turkey" on sugar and all sweeteners. Your tastes will change, but as long as you indulge, you will feel the cravings. If I have something sweet, the cravings come back for the next several days. They aren't as strong as before, but it is surprising how just a small amount of sugar sets it off.

As Dr. Joseph Mercola says, "If you stick to it, you *will* transition to burning fat, and you will enjoy reduced hunger and a dramatic reduction in cravings for sweets. And if you are like most people, you have struggled with that your entire life." [14]

Sugar – an old enemy

More about the Eskimos

In 1951, a German Doctor, Otto Schaefer, visited the Intuits in the Canadian Arctic. In some regions the Hudson Bay Company had been delivering annual boatloads of food, mainly:

- molasses (sugar)
- flour

- biscuits
- tea

However, some regions were still eating their original diet of meat, fish and fat. This was a unique opportunity to see what impact these foods had on the Inuit population.

The Inuit that were eating their traditional diets continued to be very healthy. Schaefer examined four thousand Canadian Inuit. He saw no signs of vitamin or mineral deficiencies, even with no fruits or vegetables being eaten. Amazingly, he found no lack of vitamin D, in spite of the dark winter months. He found that these diseases were nearly nonexistent:

- cardiovascular disease
- cancer
- asthma
- ulcers
- gout

- diabetes
- ulcerative colitis
- hypertension
- psychosomatic diseases

However, among the Inuit that ate the shipments of sugar and flour from the Hudson Bay Company, these diseases began to appear:

- Diabetes
- Anemia

- Tooth decay
- Chronic ear infections

In one settlement, the Iqaluit, where they were eating potato chips and drinking soft drinks, diseases were so rampant that he said it approached the level of "self-inflicted genocide." [39]

Diseases beginning in England and elsewhere

These changes were also happening in England. Between 1710 and 1770, the English began eating five times as much sugar. By 1750 sugar was the most valuable commodity in European trade, even surpassing grain. It made up one fifth of European imports. Most of this sugar came from the West Indies.

The English went from eating 4 pounds of sugar per person per year, to 20 pounds in 1790's.

What did all of this sugar do to the health in Great Britain?

Britain began to see its first cases of heart disease. As sugar increased, so did heart disease. By 1900, the average Britain was eating 80 pounds of sugar per year.

To summarize, they went from 4 pounds of sugar per person per year in 1710, to 20 ponds in 1790, to 80 pounds per year in 1900. Wow! By comparison, how much do Americans eat? In 2000, Americans were eating 150 pounds of sugar per capita (including high fructose corn syrup). Again, wow!

The other disease that began to appear was cancer, in England and elsewhere.

The same dramatic increase we saw in heart disease, we also found in cancer, as each culture went from eating its traditional foods and began to eat sugar and white flour.

And in Africa

George Prentice, a physician who studied isolated people in the Southern Central Africa in the early twentieth century, observed that as Western foods are introduced into the diet, these diseases began to appear:

- Cardiovascular disease
- Hypertension and stroke
- Cancer
- Obesity
- Diabetes
- Cavities
- Periodontal disease

- Appendicitis
- Peptic ulcers
- Diverticulitis
- Gallstones
- Hemorrhoids
- Constipation
- Varicose veins

What exactly were these foods? They were foods that would not spoil on an ocean voyage. They were primarily:

- Sugar
- Molasses

- White flour
- White rice

They were refined carbohydrates. With these foods came diseases. At that time, these diseases were called "Western diseases", or "diseases of civilization".

Dr. Richard MacKarness and low carb in 1958

When Ansel Keyes was making his pitch to have the government follow the low-fat guidelines (see section on government recommendations), there were many competing views at that time. There were people like Dr. Richard MacKarness who ran Britain's first obesity and food allergy clinic. Based on his experience in helping people lose weight, he wrote a book in 1958 called *Eat Fat and Grow Slim*. [79] He argued that it was eating carbohydrates, not excess calories, that caused weight gain.

He suggests how often we should eat certain foods. *(Italics are my additions)*:

Eat as much of these as desired:

- Meat *(This was before we were putting cattle on feed lots for their last few months)*
- Poultry
- Game
- Fish and other seafood *(This was before most fish were contaminated with mercury)*
- Dairy products *(This was before we were adding hormones, antibiotics, and pesticides to our dairy)*
- Fats and oils
- Most vegetables
- Some fruits

These foods can be eaten with moderation:

- Nuts
- Higher carb vegetables
- Fruits

These can be eaten once a day:

- Beans
- Beets
- Corn
- Potatoes
- Bananas

We should never eat these:

- Breakfast cereals
- Bread and rolls
- Biscuits and crackers
- Macaroni products, noodles, spaghetti, and other pastas
- Rice
- Jellies, jams, and preserves
- Ice cream, cakes, pies, and candy
- Sauces and gravies thickened with flour or cornstarch
- Beer
- Sweet wines and liqueurs
- Sodas (and all sweetened fizzy drinks)
- Sugar

Notice that this "never eat" list is mostly processed foods.

He suggests that we keep our carb consumption to 60 grams a day for most people, and perhaps limited to 50 grams a day for others. **Interestingly, this list of foods and carbohydrate recommendations are very similar to many of today's low-carb books.**

MacKarness also pointed out that there is an **emotional component to overeating.** He says that overeating is a result of loneliness, fear or emotional dissatisfaction, and that people are especially drawn to eating sugars and starches when they are unhappy.

So far, then, two big factors in the production of obesity have emerged.

- A defect in dealing with carbohydrates which makes a person fatten easily on an ordinary mixed diet
- Overeating, especially of sugars and starches as a result of loneliness, fear, or emotional dissatisfaction

I think MacKarness got it exactly right when he said:

"When the two factors are preset, weight is gained very rapidly. So, anyone who finds himself tempted to overeat for emotional reasons and who shows a tendency to get fat, should be careful to choose low-carbohydrate foods." [79]

Overeaters Anonymous

Interestingly, Overeaters Anonymous began about this time. Alcoholics can completely eliminate alcohol from their diet. However, we have to eat. So, some members of OA concentrated on carbohydrates, especially sugar and white flour, as the foods to stay away from. They also focus on the emotional and spiritual components of overeating.

The sugar manufacturers

The sugar manufacturers seemed very happy with the idea that fat was the food to avoid. They perpetuated this idea by telling us that all calories are the same.

The thinking goes something like this:

If all calories are the same, you may as well eat lots of sugar. After all, it is fairly low in calories. Sugar has only 48 calories per tablespoon. Not like fat. Fat is 100-120 calories per tablespoon. So, eat sugar and not fat to lose weight.

That sounds logical, but it is wrong.

It is the spiking of blood sugar (and perhaps the increase in insulin) that causes disease, (from eating foods such as sugar and flour). Unlike sugar, fat is very filling, and has no effect on blood sugar. In addition, eating sugar and flour creates cravings for these foods, so a cycle of addiction is created.

Sugar is the cause

Robert Lustig, head of an obesity clinic at UCSF, took 43 obese children and eliminated added sugar for 9 days. He didn't want them to lose weight, so they tracked what each child ate, then took out the added sugar and substituted other carbohydrates. They just wanted one thing to change (eliminating sugar), so they fed them bagels instead of sweet rolls, hot dogs instead of teriyaki chicken, etc. "We didn't give them good food. We gave them crappy food." [29] They kept them on the same number of calories. If they were losing weight, they were asked to eat more. What were the results? All of their baseline levels got better.

They all got healthier. In just 9 days.

Several measures changed, but I will address two:

- **Glucose tolerance test: down 8%.** Interestingly, although they were being fed more glucose in the form of wheat, their glucose levels went down. Why? "Because now they are insulin sensitive." [29]
- **Liver fat: down 22%.** Liver fat has been proposed as the driving force in creating many other diseases.

"We reversed their metabolic syndrome and we didn't even have to change their calories. All we did was change the food. Got rid of the sugar. That's it." [29]

Personal Note

When I was a child, my mother told me about the Inuit research. That is, in part, why she banned sugar and flour from our home. She wasn't 100% strict about this, but she would often say that sugar and flour were poison. That was 60 years ago.

This isn't new information.

Personal story about sugar

When I was 67, my youngest child had a new baby and asked me if I would like to live with him and his family and take care of the newborn. I was delighted to have that opportunity, so we all lived together for about a year.

He also had an adorable 2-year-old daughter. She loved Oreo cookies. I had not had an Oreo cookie for years, but as part of our grandma-granddaughter fun together, we ate Oreo cookies.

My knee and back began to hurt. My knee started to hurt so much that I had to walk with a cane. The doctor told me that it was an injury that would heal in a few weeks. The physical therapist told me that I had arthritis and that it would get progressively worse until I was totally disabled.

It gradually improved enough so that I could walk, but it did not go away.

After a joyful year with my son, his wife, and little granddaughters, I came home and went back on my usual diet. Immediately all of the pain went away. Wow! I was very happy about that.

Every once in a while, my knee would hurt. I would ask myself, "What did I do yesterday?" Gradually, I realized that the pattern was that I had eaten sugar the day before.

Eating sugar was making my joints hurt.

It has now been 5 years, and my knees continue to be pain-free.

Personal Story about sugar

As I approached my 70th birthday, I started to have problems with balance and vertigo. I know that many older people have balance issues. I always thought it was from taking medication, or because they didn't exercise, and their muscles were weakening.

However, I don't take any medication, and I exercise regularly.

The balance problem got progressively worse over the next nine months. I stopped using ear buds, thinking that maybe they were irritating my inner ear. That didn't help. I got an MRI to check for a brain tumor. No brain tumor. I kept trying things that I thought might be causing it. Finally, I figured it out.

It was sugar, alcohol, and anything that spiked blood sugar.

I eliminated almost all sugar, even limiting sugar from fruit. I eliminated alcohol and grains (mostly). The problem didn't disappear, but almost.

Interestingly, in the three years since this problem began, I have seen many doctors. Not one mentioned diet as a possible solution or even a contributing factor.

Occasionally, I have a glass of wine, or a dessert with sugar and flour. The balance and vertigo problems come back, and they sometimes last for several days. It doesn't take much to set it off.

Glycemic Index (GI), Glycemic Load, and Insulin Resistance

The Glycemic index (GI) is a number from 0 to 100 with pure glucose given a value of 100. The GI shows the rise of blood glucose two hours after a particular food is eaten.

Fat does not raise blood sugar. Protein contains no carbohydrate, but our bodies can convert excess protein into glucose. However, the Glycemic Index only rates carbohydrates.

The higher the blood sugar after eating a particular carbohydrate, the higher the glycemic index of that food. A low GI is 55 or less, medium is 56-69, and high is over 70.

So, how do bread and sugar rate?

The glycemic index (GI) of	
White bread	75
Whole grain bread	74
Sucrose (table sugar)	65 [80]

They are all high, but **the glycemic index of wheat is even higher than sugar.** I bet that is a surprise to many of you.

Compare to some other high GI foods:	
White rice	75-89
Rice Milk	86
Corn flakes	81
Russet Potato	72
Instant mashed potato	78
Potato chips	75
Rice crackers	87
Watermelon	76

What are some medium GI foods?

Honey	61
Soft drinks/soda	59
Popcorn	65
Brown rice	54-68
Pineapple	59
French fries	63
Raisins	64

How about some lower GI foods:

Raw apple	36
Apple juice	41
Orange	43
Orange juice	50
Banana	51
Dark chocolate	40
Beans (different varieties)	24-32
Whole fat milk	39
Soya beans	16
Soy milk	34
Corn	52
Corn tortilla	46
Dates	42
Strawberry jam/jellly	49
Yams and sweet potatoes	50

What's really low?

Artichoke	15
Asparagus	14

Bell peppers	10
Broccoli	10
Cabbage	10
Cauliflower	15
Celery	15
Green beans	14
Mushrooms	10
Onion	10 [80] [81] [82]

What about candy bars?

Mars bar	68
Snickers bar	41

Notice that wheat and white bread elevate blood sugar even more than some candy bars.

More important than the glycemic index is the **glycemic load** of the meal. All of the things eaten together at one time add up to the glycemic load. If you eat a potato along with a variety of other vegetables, and some fats, this leads to a lower glycemic load in the meal, compared to eating just the potato. A lower glycemic load keeps blood sugar from spiking.

It is interesting to note that Dale Bredesen, an expert in Alzheimer's, suggests that we only eat foods with a GI of 35 or lower. [83]

Glucose, insulin, and addiction

When we eat carbohydrates, glucose and insulin go up.
What is the problem with insulin going up?
Insulin is the hormone that allows glucose to enter the cells of the body, converting glucose to energy and to fat. The pancreas makes insulin. The higher the blood glucose, the higher the insulin level, and the more fat that is stored in the cell. Consequently, **those who eat foods with a high GI will tend to gain weight as fat. Those who eat too much protein may also have this problem.**

If we eat foods high in glucose on a regular basis, and **blood sugar is repeatedly spiking, other problems begin to occur.**

We can overwhelm the ability of the pancreas to make enough insulin. When this happens, we develop **diabetes.**

Repeated spiking of blood sugar causes **inflammation.** Ongoing inflammation is the source of many chronic diseases. These include cancer, heart disease, arthritis, MS, Alzheimer's, and many more.

If insulin is frequently spiking, we will become "**insulin resistant**". This means that insulin will start to lose its effectiveness. We need more and more insulin to do the same job. We get into a cycle of more blood glucose, more insulin, increased fat, increased insulin resistance, and on and on.

After the spike in blood sugar, there is a crash. We feel the euphoria of the rush of sugar in our bodies as the sugar is charging into our cells, but soon after we feel the crash of our blood sugar. We may feel a loss of energy, brain fog, sleepiness, and sometimes depression. And hunger. We want the euphoric rush of blood sugar again. **Sugar and wheat are addictive in this way.** The only way to get away from this addiction is to greatly reduce or eliminate everything that spikes our blood sugar. The two biggest culprits are sugar and wheat.

Instead of eating foods that spike our blood sugar, it is much healthier to eat foods that release glucose into our blood gradually over a long period of time. These are foods lower on the glycemic index scale. Foods that keep our blood sugar from spiking include fats, protein, and non-starchy vegetables, with limited amounts of whole fruits. However, it should be noted that protein also increases insulin, although not to the extent that processed carbohydrates do.

The cure for unwanted sugar cravings

What most people don't realize is that the cravings go away if we eliminate these foods. When I talk to people about changing their diet, a common response is that they cannot possibly give up sweets and/or bread. That is their addiction talking. If they gave up these things, even for one week, the cravings would most likely be reduced, and on their way to going away. There are so many delicious foods to replace sweets and bread.

We have been on a low-fat craze for at least 50 years. Fat is now considered healthy (not by everyone). Replace sugar and wheat with delicious protein and healthy fats. Imagine eating meat, such as grass-fed ribeye steaks, pasture-fed eggs, healthy bacon, cheese and sour cream from grass-fed cows, wild-caught salmon, avocados, nuts and seeds, and a range of organic vegetables cooked in animal fats. These foods can be a healthy and delicious alternative to sugar and flour.

> ### Challenge

> If you don't believe this, I challenge you to try it. Give up added sugar and wheat for one week.
> I predict that:
> • The thought of giving them up will be harder than actually doing it.
> • You will be shocked at how much better you feel.
> • Your cravings for sweets and wheat products will be reduced.
> • You will not feel as hungry.
> • You may lose weight, maybe even easily.
> • Your long-term illnesses may begin to mysteriously disappear.

Try it!

Wheat and Other Grains -- Enemy #2?

"People are usually shocked when I tell them that whole wheat bread increases blood sugar to a higher level than sucrose."
--P.R. Shewry [84]

"Aside from some extra fiber, eating two slices of whole wheat bread is really little different, and often worse, than drinking a can of sugar-sweetened soda or eating a sugary candy bar."
--William Davis, M.D. [85]

But, wait. **Isn't whole wheat supposed to be good for us?** Let's take a look.

Grains and Other Carbohydrates

Wheat. Wheat is a huge problem in the American diet. Why do I say this?

- **We eat way too much of it, leaving little room in our diets for the healthy foods we should be eating.** [85]
- **Wheat spikes blood sugar more than sugar.**
- It has been **altered so much** that the nutritional content has changed radically. Today's wheat has very little nutrition and much more gluten.
- It is usually **sprayed with glyphosate** at the end of growing to kill it quickly to make it ready for harvest. This leaves most wheat with poison residue on it.
- Many people have issues with **gluten**, even if they are not aware of it. Wheat and gluten are two of the most common allergies.

There are so many reasons to avoid wheat. Let's look at these in more detail.

Wheat used to be a tall plant. We have changed wheat so that now it is a **short stalk with a very large heavy seed.** We now produce much more wheat per acre, but what are we eating? Today's wheat has a much higher gluten content with different nutrition. We don't really know what this product does to us because it is so new as a food. It does seem odd to me that we are willing to eat a large part of our diet as something that is a Frankenstein (meaning human-made) food.

Most people probably don't realize how much wheat they eat. Wheat has very little nutrition or fiber. That doesn't leave much room for the range of nutrition that we are supposed to be eating in a day, such as colorful fruits and vegetables and healthy fats.

Sadly, the government food pyramid encouraged Americans to eat primarily wheat products each day. This was terrible advice. Most Americans are used to eating large amounts of wheat at every meal. Americans have cereal, toast, or pancakes for breakfast, sandwiches or pizza for lunch, bread with dinner, or a bun with their burger, then cake or cookies for dessert. **We are simply eating way too much of a very unhealthy food.**

Very few people eat wheat as a whole grain. Instead, we buy wheat already ground and processed and baked into products for us. These usually have "preservatives, pesticides to keep insects away, chemical substances to prevent it absorbing moisture, color and flavor improvers and softeners, just to mention a few." [44]

Grains and glycemic index (GI)

Wheat. Whole wheat bread has a glycemic index of 74 (That's high).

Oats. Some researchers say to avoid all grains, including oats, primarily because it spikes blood sugar. Others say it is beneficial. Benefits of eating oats may include:

- Reducing risk of coronary artery disease
- Lowering levels of cholesterol
- Reducing risk of colorectal cancer (although recent research does not support this). [77]
- **Glycemic index of oats is 59.**

Rice. Avoid white rice due to the high glycemic index. Also, it has very little nutrition. Brown rice is better because it has more nutrition but it still has a high GI. Wild rice is a good choice (really a grass, not a grain). **Glycemic index is 75-89.**

However, Chinese have been eating white rice as a large part of their diet, and until recently, have been slim and healthy on this diet. The Chinese started to become obese and unhealthy when they added sugar to their diets. [77]

Quinoa. It is actually a seed, not a grain. However, it is a starchy seed, as opposed to an oily seed (like most seeds). This is why it is often put in the grain category.

It is unusual in that it has all of the essential amino acids (complete protein). However, it can raise blood sugar if eaten in larger quantities. If eaten with low GI foods, like vegetables, it can be an acceptable food to eat. It is a great substitute for grains or rice. I find that it has a very appealing flavor compared to most other grains.

It has a relatively low GI of 53.

Pasta. This is usually made from wheat, and can spike blood sugar. I recommend not eating it, or eating it infrequently in small amounts. However, some people really love pasta, so if you are going to eat it, I recommend not eating wheat pasta, but instead eating pasta made from quinoa, or a quinoa and corn mix or pasta made from edamame.

GI is 43-58, depending on the type of grain.

What about using other flours instead of wheat? There are ancient grains such as amaranth, teff, buckwheat, millet, rye, and spelt. I think these are preferable to wheat because they are fairly unchanged. They are the grains of our ancestors. However, if they are ground into flour, they still spike blood sugar in a similar way to wheat. Wheat, rye, and barley are the grains that contain gluten.

Flax seed flour. I recommend using flax seed as a flour in baking. It is not a grain. It has healthy fats, and has a low **glycemic index of only 32**. I think that it makes a very tasty flour.

Potatoes. Potatoes are not grains, but they are a starchy carbohydrate, and because they are eaten in such quantities, they deserve mention. Americans eat an average 125 pounds of potatoes per year per person, or about one potato a day.

Americans eat:

- **4.5 billion pounds of French fries.**
- **6.7 billion pounds of potatoes made into potato chips**
- **75 million pounds of Tater Tots [86]**

These are eaten without the skin, which has most of the fiber and nutrition.

If you want to be healthy, eliminate or at least minimize the amount of potatoes you eat.

Try eating other root vegetables, such as parsnips, beets, radishes, rutabagas, or turnips. Even eating more unusual varieties of potatoes (such as fingerling) are better than the russet potato.

And never deep-fry anything.

Potatoes have a GI of 72-111, depending on the kind.

In summary, with regard to all grains and potatoes, we are eating

simply too much of these. We should be eating about 80% of our food as non-starchy vegetables, by volume, and up to 70 % of our food as healthy fats, as measured in calories. So, lots of fresh colorful organic vegetables and lots of healthy fats.

Are we doing that? No. We are primarily eating sugar, grains (mostly wheat), and unhealthy fats. No wonder we are so unhealthy and overweight!

Seed Oils May be the Worst of All

"They are poisons, plain and simple"
--Chris Knobbe, M.D. [11]

Why are we so sick? Some researchers think that sugar is the main problem (Gary Taubes), some think that it is grains (David Perlmutter), and some think that it is seed and bean oils, commonly called "vegetable oils". The main proponent of this is Chris Knobbe.

Dr. Knobbe says that 80% of our diseases of civilization are because of vegetable oils and trans fats, and only 15% is due to sugar, and only 5% is because of refined wheat. [11] Let's take a look at why he says this.

Are seed oils even worse than sugar?

A study of 195,000 participants, published in the British Medical Journal, concluded that seed oils increased mortality more than sugar when their intake exceeded 6-7% of calories. Most people eat more seed oils than this. In fact, Australians average 13% of their calories as seed oils.

Eating saturated fats leads to a much lower overall mortality than eating seed oils. [87]

Why do we think that seed oils are healthy when they are really so deadly?

In 1977, the U.S. government started making recommendations about what Americans should eat.

The government recommended that we:

- **Reduce our intake of fat overall to 30 per cent of calories.**

- **Reduce our intake of saturated fat to 10% of total calories.**
- **Eat vegetable oils instead of saturated fats.**

These recommendations were never based on research or science, according to Zoe Harcombe, Ph.D. [88]

These recommendations continue to this day, with the most recent guidelines in 2020 suggesting that we continue to keep our saturated fat intake to no more than 10% of calories.

In order to **make packaged food taste good without saturated fats,** food manufacturers started putting sugar in their products. Consequently, instead of saturated fats, **we started eating large amounts of sugar, refined grains, and vegetable oils.**

These recommendations have been a miserable failure. [14] Eating these foods has caused an explosion of health problems.

For example,

- **Diabetes** has increased from 5.19 million in 1978 to 22.3 million in 2013. [89] **It has quadrupled in only 35 years.**
- **Obesity.** In 1970 only about one in six people were obese. Now it is about one out of three adults.

Many **healthy oils** come from plants, including:

- Coconut oil
- Olive oil
- Walnut oil
- Avocado oil

However, there are also unhealthy oils. These come from seeds, beans, and grains. [90] These are:

- Canola
- Soybean
- Corn
- Cottonseed
- Rapeseed
- Grapeseed
- Sunflower
- Safflower
- Rice bran

Trans fats are the worst of all, but they have been largely eliminated from our diets.

Why are these unhealthy oils a problem?

1. **They are unstable.** The main reason seed oils are so toxic is that they easily oxidize, primarily from light and heat. This means they go rancid easily, creating inflammation and free radicals, which can cause cell damage. These oxidized products can enter our organs. It is damage to the liver that can cause insulin resistance. [90] [87]

2. **They have too many omega 6's**, which leads to an imbalance of omega 3's and 6's. Ideally, we should have approximately a 1:1 balance of 3's to 6's. Since we eat too many of these unhealthy oils, many Americans have a 10:1 or even a 25:1 ratio. This makes it very difficult for our bodies to use the omega 3's. The omega 6's crowd out the omega 3's. Keep in mind that both omega 3 and omega 6 are essential to our health, but we are getting too many omega 6's if we eat seed oils. [90]

3. **They are highly refined.** Vegetable oils, in their natural state, don't taste and smell very good, and most of them aren't even digestible. In order to make them at all edible, they need to be refined, getting rid of their taste and smell. **This is done at high heat, and harsh chemical solvents must be used.**

4. They are often made from **genetically modified (GMO) crops.** These may have residual poisons that could damage your microbiome (the healthy bacteria living in your gut).

Omega 3's are found in coldwater fish, pasture-raised meats, pasture-raised eggs, flax, nuts, and chia seeds.

Omega 6's are found in factory farmed meats, and eggs from grain-fed chickens (because they eat foods high in omega 6's).

Mostly, our high **omega 6's come from eating the seed, bean, and grain oils**, also called "industrial oils" (because they are made in factories similar to petroleum oil factories). [39]

Let's look at how canola oil is made.

Canola oil comes from the rapeseed plant. By itself, it is not edible as a food. For many years, we used this oil for industrial purposes. In order to make it into a "food", it needs to be processed at high heat with a harsh chemical solvent called hexane.

"This oil is not recognized in the body as food. And it's questionable whether it's even remotely fit for human consumption. And what is true for canola oil goes for all the other industrial oils too, especially soy oil, which has also deceptively been sold to us as a health food." [90]

How is cottonseed oil made?

Deodorized cottonseed oil, known as Wesson oil, appeared on the food market in 1899. At that time, the majority of foods that Americans ate were whole, unprocessed, and locally grown. They were also organic, as synthetic fertilizers and pesticides had not yet been introduced. [14]

Cottonseed oil began as a waste product of the cotton industry. Initially, it was used to make soap and as fuel for lamps. Cottonseed oil, in its natural state, is cloudy, with a red tint due to the presence of a toxic element called gossypol. An article in Popular Science said, "What was garbage in 1860 was fertilizer in 1870, cattle feed in 1880, and table food and many things else in 1890." [91]

One of the problems with all polyunsaturated fats is that they are very unstable and go rancid easily. In 1909, Edwin Kayser developed a process for making unstable liquid fats into solid and stable fats. This process was called hydrogenation. Hydrogenated cottonseed oil looked like lard (pig fat), the most popular cooking oil at that time. Proctor and Gamble decided to sell hydrogenated cottonseed oil as a food, and called it Crisco. [14]

Proctor and Gamble did an amazing marketing campaign, and successfully increased sales from 2.6 million pounds in 1912 to 60 million pounds just four years later. [92]

"The advent of Crisco on the shelves and pantries across America kicked off what is probably the era of the greatest chronic degeneration in human health!" [92]

Healthy oils

Healthy plant oils are often made by just cold pressing. For example, extra-virgin olive oil isn't exposed to high heat and harsh solvents. It is simply ground up and put in a press.

However, even olive oil and fish oil can go bad fairly quickly. [87]

The safest oils are from fresh meat (lard and tallow), butter, and eating fresh fish.

Coconut oil

Coconut oil has a high percentage of saturated fat. Is coconut oil healthy?

The inhabitants of the Tokelau Islands (between Hawaii and Australia) were studied from the 1960's to the 1980's. What do they eat?

- Coconut (54-62% of calories)
- Fish
- Starchy tubers
- Fruit

Coconut oil is 91-94.5% saturated fat. Their total diet is 53% fat with 48% saturated fat.

In 1982 men between 40-69 were studied. They had no heart attacks, no obesity, and no diabetes. They were extremely healthy.

Saturated fats in coconut oil does not seem to be a problem.

> **Take away on seed oils**

- **Highly processed vegetable oils are toxic to our bodies, and are to be avoided. A large part of our calories come from these toxic oils that provide very little nutrition. No wonder we are so sick!**

Processed foods

Processed foods are 63-74% of our diets.

This breaks down into:

- 32% vegetable oil
- 17% refined wheat
- 21% sugar
- Trans fats are now down to only 1% [11]

Said another way, these 3 foods make up 63% of the American diet:

- **Sugar**
- **White flour (today flour is 20% of the world's diet)**
- **Vegetable oils**

All of these have almost no nutrition. That leaves only about 26% to 37% of our food from which to get our nutrition, and much of that has residual poison from glyphosate (roundup), or other pesticides or herbicides.

When were the elements of processed foods introduced?

Sugar	1822
Cottonseed oil	1866
White flour	1880
Crisco (trans fats)	1911

We had all of the processed foods available to eat by 1911. [11]

How long have we known that processed foods were toxic?

We have known for at least 100 years that these foods were unhealthy. In 1918 Elmer B McCollum wrote a book called *The Newer Knowledge of Nutrition: The Use of Food for the Preservation of Vitality and Health.* It covers thousands of animal studies. One of the studies compared rats eating different kinds of fat. [93] One group of rats ate 5% cottonseed oil with the other rats eating 1.5% butterfat. The rats on the cottonseed oil grew to 60% of normal size and lived about half as long and were sickly. The rats on the butterfat were normal size, healthy, and lived twice as long. Why? **Dr. Knobbe says that it was the lack of fat-soluble vitamins, A, D, and K2. Plant oils do not have these vitamins.**

McCollum wrote, back in 1918, that the diet must contain several things. "One of these is associated with certain fats, and is especially abundant in butter fat, egg yolk fats, and the fats of glandular organs such as the liver and kidney but is not found in any fats or oils of vegetable origin." [93]

Weston A. Price wrote about the dangers of these foods in 1939. He said that Western diseases were driven by these foods.

The dangers of these foods were known and well-documented. However, as a country, we ignored this information. [11]

History of consumption of "vegetable oils".

Vegetable oils were about 2% of our diet until 1909. [94] **Now they are 32% of our calories. About 20% of our calories come from just**

soybean oil. Soybean oil is in almost all processed foods. [46]

Again, one third of our calories are from vegetable oils that are highly processed and have very little nutrition.

In 1900, 99% of our fats came from animal fats. What were these?

- Tallow (rendered beef or mutton fat)
- Suet (raw beef or mutton fat around loin and kidneys)
- Lard (pork fat)
- Beef fat

By 2005, 86% of our oils came from vegetable oils. [11]

The formal dietary guidelines from the government were introduced in 1977. Our vegetable oil consumption continued going up. This has been happening all over the world, not just America. [11]

Comparing the development of diseases to the addition of processed foods to our diets. [11]

Heart disease

- **In Boston in 1811 there were no heart disease deaths reported.** However, there were 25 sudden deaths reported, so perhaps 2.6% of deaths could have been heart failure.
- In the entire 1800's there were only 8 papers worldwide reporting heart disease.
- Sir William Osler, a physician at Johns Hopkins, reports 6 cases of angina in the previous 21 years. No heart attacks (1897).
- In 1900 12.5% of deaths were due to "heart disease" but these deaths were cardiac valvular (from syphilis or rheumatic fever), not coronary heart disease (arteries clogging). (Jones)
- In 1912 we have the first known case of heart disease confirmed with autopsy evidence. (John Harry)
- By 1930, heart attacks were the leading cause of death
- **Now it is one in three (32% of deaths)**

Cancer

- **In 1811, 1 in 188 people died of cancer.**
- By 1900 5.8% of deaths were due to cancer. That is 1 in 17.
- **By 2010, 31.1% deaths are due to cancer. Almost one third of deaths.**

Diabetes

In the 1800's it is very rare.

- **1935, it is .37%**
- 1960 it is .91%
- 1991 it is 2.97%,
- 2010 it is 6.95%
- **2015 it is 9.4%**

That is a 25-fold increase in 80 years

Obesity

- **1880   1.2%**
- 1960   13%
- 1980   13%
- 1988   23%
- 1999   30%
- 2005   34%
- 2011   35%
- **2015   39.8%**

This is a 33-fold increase in 150 years.

Age-related Macular degeneration (AMD)

- **1851-1930,** there were fewer than 50 cases reported worldwide in the entire 80 years (**one in many thousands**).
- **By 2020,** there are 196,000,000 cases worldwide, and **almost one in three for those over 75).**

Almost every advisory group in the United States (government food pyramid, American Heart Association, American Diabetes Association, American Cancer Society, etc.) has been recommending that we decrease our intake of saturated fats and increase our intake of carbohydrates and vegetable oils.

Knobbe suggests that this recommendation has been part, perhaps a major part, of the obesity and health crisis we are now in.

Take Away

• Our biggest killers are sugar, flour, and highly processed "vegetable" oils. They make up 63 per cent of the American diet, mostly in the form of processed and packaged foods. They have calories but very little nutrition. They are all to be minimized or eliminated.

• As these foods are introduced into our diets, the rates of diseases such as heart disease, cancer, diabetes, obesity, and macular degeneration dramatically increase. This is happening all around the world when "Western foods" are introduced.

Chapter 5

Getting It So Wrong

Farming allowed civilization to develop.

We started farming about 10,000 years ago. Before that, we were all hunter/gatherers, and the human population was very small, about 5 million in the entire world.

Farming allowed us to grow an abundance of food and store food. In 1900, just over 100 years ago, the world population was 1.6 billion. In the United States, 38% of the work force was still farmers. It has only been since we developed machines that just a few people can grow the food for almost everyone else.

Today, only 2% of the U.S. work force is farmers and ranchers. It has only been the last hundred years that we have had such an abundance of food. For the first time in human history, we have food from all over the world, all year round.

This has allowed the human population to explode.

From 1900 to 1950, the population went from 1.6 billion to 2 billion. Now, in 2020, it is 7.64 billion. (U.S. Census Bureau)

Government Subsidies

Before WWII, there were sometimes food shortages. There was the dust bowl, the depression, and food rationing during WWII. After WWII, the nation went on a campaign to increase food production. The government started heavily subsidizing certain foods. This is where the money goes:

Meat and dairy	63%
Grains	20%
Sugar, starch, oil, alcohol	15%
Nuts and legumes	2%
Fruits and vegetables	1%

Because of government subsidies, some foods are really cheap to grow. Food manufacturers put these ingredients in their foods. That is one reason why high fructose corn syrup is so prevalent in processed foods. It's cheap.

The factory farms started taking over small family farms. Farming became a huge industry. Food became a commodity. It was plentiful and cheap. This project of making abundant food has been a resounding success.

But wait! Food is not just a commodity. Lots of cheap food is fine as long as it also does the job of supplying enough nutrition for us to be healthy. We need more than just calories from food. Sadly, much of our nutrition got lost along the way.

Herbicides and pesticides kill the soil

Healthy soil is rich with microorganisms. There are more microbes in one third cup of healthy soil, than there are people on earth! Soil microorganisms include: bacteria, fungi, algae, protozoa, insects, spiders, nematodes and worms.

On large factory farms, we add fertilizer back into the soil to try to give our food some nutrition, but that adds only a few nutrients. Therefore, most of **our food has very little nutrition.**

Another thing we like to have from our food is taste. That has also largely gotten lost along the way. We have been selecting produce for shelf-life. In the process, we have lost much of the flavor.

But you say that you love the food you are eating. That's because it full of salt, sugar, processed fats, and chemicals to enhance the flavor. You rarely get to taste the actual food.

Those of you who are older probably remember what tomatoes used to taste like. I remember that they were so good we would eat them like apples. They were sweet and delicious. They would go bad in a few days. Now they have very little taste and will sit on the counter for a month without going bad. The skin will wrinkle, but the tomato doesn't change much.

Fortunately, there are still people who grow food who care about taste and nutrition. Your best source may be the local farmer's markets, where, in most cities, there is an abundance of locally grown organic produce.

Whole Foods and Costco also have a good range of organic delicious food. In addition, most groceries here in California have a fresh organic produce section.

In conclusion, we are really good at producing an abundance of cheap food. However, we have lost nutrition and taste along the way. And, sadly, we are also adding an array of poisons to our food.

Ansel Keyes starts the low-fat trend

Ansel Keyes was a very popular and influential physician during and after WWII. He developed "K-rations" for the military during WWII. "K" is for Keyes.

After the war, he published a study showing that high cholesterol is associated with heart disease. He graphed incidence of heart attacks and cholesterol consumption by country. However, he only included the 7 countries that supported his theory, not the 22 total that would not have supported his ideas.

He was instrumental in starting the United States on the "low-fat diet" that has dominated our eating for more than 50 years.

Many researchers disagreed with him, but he was very persuasive, and succeeded in directing government policies.

The truth is that in many countries in Europe, especially France, the more saturated fat eaten, the lower the heart attack rate -- just the opposite of what he concluded.

He said that it is eating fat that makes people fat. That seems believable. However, it just happens to be wrong.

Framingham Heart Study supports low-fat

Another reason we went in the wrong direction was the Framingham Heart Study. This was a cardiovascular study on the residents of Framingham, Massachusetts. It began in 1948 with 5,209 adults and is now studying the third generation of residents.

This study found many important risk factors for heart disease. The primary findings included:

- Cigarette smoking, high blood pressure, and obesity increase risk
- Exercise and high HDL cholesterol reduce risk

But it also found, incorrectly, that high cholesterol is a risk factor. This is one more reason we began to believe that cholesterol increases the risk for heart disease.

Mann, one of the original researchers of Framingham, went on to collect data on food consumption from one thousand subjects. When he collated them in 1960, he found that eating saturated fat had no relationship to heart disease.

Thirty years after the project started, the researchers found that once men passed the age of 47, it didn't make any difference if his cholesterol was low or high. They concluded that lowering cholesterol was only important for men with a history of heart disease who were under 47.

In addition, in the 30-year follow-up report, they found that "for each 1% mg/dl drop of cholesterol there was an 11% increase in coronary and total mortality." [95] **Not a decrease, as would be expected, but an increase in mortality from lowering cholesterol!** This is exactly the opposite of what would be expected from the previous published findings. Oops!

Sadly, these later findings were ignored. The medical profession, the researchers, the pharmaceutical industry and the government had already made up their minds. They did not want to deal with facts that contradicted their beliefs. Not everyone, of course, but the trend was set.

Later, 44 years after the study began, the director of the study, William Castelli, M.D. wrote the following, published in the Archives of Internal Medicine:

"We found that people who ate the most cholesterol, ate the most saturated fat, and ate the most calories weighed the least and were the most physically active." [33]

A biochemist, George Mann, M.D., who helped develop the Framingham Heart Study, later said that the idea that cholesterol is a risk factor in heart disease is "the greatest scam ever perpetrated on the American public." [33]

For a very thorough review of this part of history, I suggest you read *The Big Fat Surprise* by Nina Teicholz.

Obesity in America.

We have not always been this fat. In fact, it is a relatively new development. When did this explosion of diseases and obesity really take off?

In 1977, United States Senate Select Committee on Nutrition and Human Needs, with George McGovern as its chairman, released recommendations about what Americans should eat. These guidelines included:

- Carbohydrates should be increased to 55-60% of calories.
- Fat should be decreased from 40 to 30% of calories, and only 10% of total calories should come from saturated fats.

Americans did what they thought they were supposed to do. Refined grain consumption increased, sugar consumption increased, and fat consumption decreased. The result? Obesity began to climb.

We have been told that the way to lose weight is to "eat less and exercise more". Most of us have tried this. Does it work?

We have been told that if we eat fewer calories, we will lose weight. Initially, this does happen, but then our weight loss stops. Why? One reason is that our metabolism changes to adjust to the decrease in calories coming in. See chapter on Ideal Weight.

U.S. Dietary guidelines

Dr. Joseph Mercola summarizes it well.

"The American medical community and mainstream media began advising people to stop consuming the butter, lard, and bacon they'd been eating for centuries, replacing them with bread, pasta, margarine, low-fat dairy, and vegetable oil." These recommendations have **"actually fueled the problem it aimed to treat. No one knows for sure just how many premature deaths have resulted from this low-fat diet recommendation, but my guess is that number is easily into the hundreds of millions."** [14]

Government Food Recommendations

Americans have been following the government food recommendation since 1977, when they began. The government recommendations were never based on research or science. They were always based on opinions and theories. The pharmaceutical companies and the food manufacturers pay influential people to make recommendations that will support their industries. That is how the government recommendations are developed. [96] [88]

I discovered there is a large body of solid research that does tell us what we should be eating in order to stay healthy. The conclusions from this research are not what we are being told by the healthcare system or the government, but they do exist.

In addition, this information is not new. We have known what is healthy to eat for a very long time.

These government recommendations are clearly not working. We are getting fatter and sicker as the years go by. However, in spite of the research that is in direct contradiction to the government recommendations, the American Medical Association (AMA), the American Diabetic Association (ADA), and the American Heart Association (AHA) and the American Cancer Society (ACS) are all in general agreement with the government recommendations.

This is a huge problem. I think it is important to know what these recommendations are, and how these recommendations differ from the scientific research. Let's start with looking at these government recommendations.

What are they?

We have probably all seen the government food recommendations, sometimes shown as a pyramid or a plate. The most recent one just came out for 2020-2025. I thought that perhaps because there has been so much solid research which contradicts the government recommendations, that they might have changed their thinking. But sadly, the new recommendations are very similar to the previous recommendations. Our new government recommendations are as follows. *My comments are in italics.*

- **"Vegetables of all types,** –dark green, red and orange, beans, peas, and lentils, starchy, and other vegetables." 2.5 cups. *Note that no distinction is made between starchy vegetables, such as potatoes and beans, and non-starchy vegetables, such as broccoli and onions. This includes canned vegetables that have very little nutrition.*
- **"Fruits,** especially whole fruit." 2 cups. *Note that fruits high in sugar, such as pineapple, are not differentiated from low-sugar fruits, such as blueberries. This includes fruit juice which spikes blood sugar, and canned fruit that has very little nutritional value.*
- **"Grains,** at least half of which are whole grain." 6 ounces. *Still encouraging us to eat grains. Examples they give are 5 slices of bread, or 5 ounces of ready-to eat cereal, or 2.5 cups of pasta. All of these have very little nutrition, spike blood sugar, and increase insulin.*
- **"Dairy,** including fat-free or low-fat milk, yogurt, and cheese, and/or lactose-free versions and fortified soy beverages and yogurt as alternatives." 3 cups. *Still limiting fat in milk. This includes 3 cups of milk, in spite of the fact that 75% of the world has a problem digesting lactose (see section on our ancestors).*
- **"Protein** foods, including lean meats, poultry, and eggs, seafood, beans, peas, and lentils, and nuts, seeds and soy products." 5.5 ounces. *Still discouraging saturated fats in meats.*
- **"Oils,** including vegetable oils and oils in food, such as seafood

and nuts." 27 grams. *Still encouraging vegetable oils.*

In addition to foods that the government says we should eat, **these are the foods that should be limited,** according to the 2020-2025 guidelines. *My comments are in italics.*

- **"Added sugars**—Less than 10 percent of calories per day starting at age 2. Avoid foods and beverages with added sugar for those younger than age 2." *No amount of added sugar is good, at any age.*
- **"Saturated fat** – less than 10 percent of calories per day starting at age 2." *Still limiting saturated fat. What about before age 2? Mother's milk is high in saturated fat, depending on her diet. In a study of Danish mothers, the average milk fat content was 3.9 percent (similar to whole milk) with the range between 1.8 percent (similar to low-fat milk), and 8.9 percent (similar to table cream). At 3.9%, the saturated fat in milk is 47.2% of calories. [97] "The higher fat is more desirable, of course, for the developing infant." [98] So, suddenly at age 2, saturated fat is no longer healthy, and should go from the average in mother's milk of 47.2% of calories to less than 10%? Unfortunately, Americans have switched to eating unhealthy vegetable oils instead.*
- **"Sodium** -- Less than 2,300 milligrams per day – and even less for children younger than age 14." *See section on sodium. The government recommendation does not agree with current research.*
- **"Alcoholic beverages** – Adults of legal drinking age can choose not to drink, or to drink in moderation by limiting intake to 2 drinks or less in a day for men and 1 drink or less in a day for women, when alcohol is consumed. Drinking less is better for health than drinking more. There are some adults who should not drink alcohol, such women who are pregnant." *Alcohol is processed like sugar, has little or no nutritional value, and can cause damage to our bodies. I wish the research said that drinking alcohol is unhealthy, but it actually says that 1-2 drinks is correlated with living longer. [1]*

What are the problems with these recommendations?

Dr. Sten Ekberg does an excellent job of analyzing some of these government guidelines. He points out some of the problems with these recommendations. What does he say?

The guidelines suggest two cups of fruit per day consisting of "fresh, frozen, canned, and dried fruits and 100% fruit juices." [99] Dr. Ekberg says that if you eat a combination of these fruits, in two cups, there are approximately **75 grams of sugar.** *Yes, it is a more natural form of sugar than table sugar, but it is still sugar.* [100] *If 2 cups of dried fruit is eaten, like dates, the sugar content is much higher.*

The government guidelines say to eat three cups of non-fat dairy per day. According to the guidelines, "cream, sour cream, and cream cheese are not included." [99] Dr. Ekberg states that the fat is the only thing that would slow down the insulin response of dairy. With only protein and sugar (lactose), and no fat to slow it down, the body creates a large insulin response. He says that three cups of dairy per day is about **40 grams of sugar.** [100]

The government does acknowledge that table sugar is not good for us. However, **they allow a daily added sugar intake (beyond dairy and fruit) of 10% of total calories** [99] On a 2,000-calorie diet, that is 200 calories of sugar, or **50 grams of sugar.** *That is about 12 teaspoons of sugar!*

If we add up the government recommendations for sugar consumption, we get:

- **75 grams from fruit**
- **40 grams from dairy**
- **50 grams from added sugar**
- **For a total of 165 grams of sugar.**

In addition, the government recommends that on a 2,000-calorie diet, we eat a total of 300 grams of carbohydrates. This is an extremely high number. You might think that "complex carbs" like rice, pasta and potatoes, are safe to eat (as the government suggests) but they are very quickly broken down into glucose (sugar). It only takes about 10-15 minutes. Consequently, they are really no healthier than table sugar. [100]

Dr. Ekberg concludes by saying that we should do the opposite of what the government guidelines say. We should be eating healthy fats to slow down our blood sugar and to help us feel full, and we should avoid sugars and starchy carbohydrates which drive up our insulin.

In Chapter 2, I talked about lowering my total carbohydrate intake for the day to under 50, or even under 30, to lose weight. The government recommendations, according to Dr.Ekberg's math, lead to a total caroohydrate intake of 465 grams of carbs. No wonder our insulin is out of control, and we are getting fatter and sicker!

Cigarette manufacturers -- role model for hiding the truth

Lung cancer was once a very rare disease. In the late 1800's, mechanization of cigarette machines, combined with mass marketing, helped cause a global lung cancer epidemic. It was clear by the 1940's and 1950's that cigarettes were the cause of the disease. However, cigarette manufacturers launched a campaign to deny this through very effective propaganda, such that in 1960 only one-third of all US doctors believed that cigarettes caused cancer. [101]

The pharmaceutical companies and the food manufacturers have been doing their best to follow the tobacco companies' example to keep the truth from us. [76]

What should the government recommendations be?

If the government based their food recommendations on science instead of opinions, I suggest that they might look something like this:

• Eliminate or greatly reduce all forms of sugar from our diet, including artificial sweeteners.
• Eliminate or greatly reduce all grain products from our diet, even whole wheat.
• Eat healthy saturated animal fat, or other healthy oils (such as coconut oil, olive oil, and avocado oil) instead of seed and bean oils.
• Make sure your vitamin D level is high enough. Get sun on your skin, eat food rich in vitamin D, or take a supplement (see section on Vitamin D).

- Most of the food you eat should be non-starchy vegetables (by volume).
- Use some form of fasting (giving your body time without food in your stomach, at least 12 hours per day) We may need up to 16-20 hours per day of fasting if we want excellent results, at least on some days. However, fasting is not appropriate for everyone, such as growing children or pregnant women.
- Eliminate or greatly reduce processed foods (foods that contain sugar, vegetable oil, and/or flour).
- Do not eat animals that have been fed GMO corn and soy (that is most meat available in the grocery). Instead, eat animals that have been grass-fed (beef), or pasture-fed (chickens and eggs), and/or have been eating organic food.
- Eat organic food whenever possible.

Take Away

- Factory farming has allowed us to make abundant cheap food. However, food is more than a commodity. Nutrition and taste also matter.
- The government food recommendations have sent us in the wrong direction. We are fatter and sicker than ever.
- We need to change the way we eat by eliminating all artificial ingredients, all poisons, and adding organic real foods to our diets.

Chapter 6

Longevity

Blue Zones of the world

Dan Buettner wrote a best-selling book *The Blue Zones,* in which he describes 5 areas of the world where people live the longest. People in the blue zones are the most likely to live past 100 (In the US today, the life expectancy is about 78.93 years). [102] [103]

Where Are the World's Blue Zones?

- **Sardinia, Italy.** The mountainous region of a small island off the coast of Italy.
- **Ikaria, Greece.** An Island eight miles off the coast of Turkey
- **Okinawa, Japan.** An Island that has the world's longest-lived women. It is not the whole island, but just a small group that lives in the mountains.
- **Nicoya Peninsula, Costa Rica.**
- **The Seventh-day Adventists in Loma Linda, California**

The people in these blue zones are different from each other in many ways. They live in different areas of the world. They are different races, different nationalities, and different religions. So, what do they have in common?

In another book by Dan Buettner, *The Blue Zone Solution*, he described **9 commonalities** in these Blue Zones. What are they?

- **Move Naturally.** They garden, and do lots of walking.
- **Purpose.** They have a reason for getting up in the morning. Research has shown that having a sense of purpose adds up to 7 years of life expectancy.
- **Downshift.** All of the Blue Zone groups have a ritual for downshifting. The Okinawans practice ancestor veneration, the Adventists pray, the Ikarians take a nap, and Sardinians do happy hour.
- **80% rule.** The Okinawans stop eating when they are 80% full. They eat their smallest meal in the afternoon or evening, then they don't eat after that.
- **Plant-based diet.** The one commonality in all of the groups is that they eat beans, about 1 cup a day. They eat very little meat, maybe 5 times a month and only 3-4 oz. They all primarily eat fresh vegetables.
- **Alcohol.** All of the Blue Zones drink alcohol, even some Adventists. Moderate drinkers outlive nondrinkers. The limit is 1-2 glasses per day.
- **Born to the right group.** The cultures of these 5 groups support healthy behaviors. Research shows that smoking, obesity, happiness, and even loneliness are contagious.
- **Community.** All but 5 of the 263 centenarians they interviewed belonged to a **faith-based community**. It didn't matter what faith. Research shows that attending faith-based services 4-10 times per month **could add 4-14 years to your life.**
- **Families first.** They keep **grandparents** in the home. This not only adds years to the grandparents' lives, but the children in these homes are healthier. They commit to a **life partner** (adding up to 3 years of life expectancy), and they invest in their children with time and love. [98]

They not only live longer, they are healthy right up to the end of their lives. They have a significantly lower risk of heart attacks, strokes, cancer, osteoporosis, Alzheimer's and dementia.

What do people in these Blue Zones eat?

Ikaria, Greece

Greens	17 percent by weight
Vegetables	20
Fruits	16
Legumes	11
Potatoes	9
Olive Oil	6
Fish	6
Meat	5
Pasta	5
Sweets	4
Grains	1

All fresh plant food (greens, vegetables, fruits, legumes, potatoes, and grains) accounts for 74% of the diet. That just leaves meat, fish, pasta and sweets and olive oil with 20%.

Fifty per cent of the diet is fat if we count the food by calories and half of that is olive oil.

Okinawa, Japan

The Okinawans have a rather odd diet. Almost 70% of it is sweet potatoes. Here it is:

Sweet Potatoes	67 percent by weight
Rice	12
Other vegetables	9
Legumes	6
Other grains	3
Fish, meat, poultry	2
Other foods	1

This is about 98% fresh plants!

Interestingly, in a later book, *The Blue Zone Solution,* Beuttner describes what happened when fast food hit the Okinawan population. [1] Sweet potatoes dropped from 67% to 5% of the diet, they doubled their rice consumption, grains increased from 3 to 23%, meat, fish and eggs went from 2 to 15%.

Not surprisingly, their health suffered. Cancers of the lung, breast, and colon almost doubled.

Sardinia, Italy

Grains	47 percent by weight
Dairy	26
Vegetables	12
Meat, fish, poultry	5
Legumes	4
Sweets and added sugars	3
Added fats	2
Fruits	1

Now it is grains that dominate the diet, primarily flat bread made from durum wheat. They also use barley in soups or ground into flour and made into bread. Barley is the food most highly associated with living to 100 among Sardinian men. It is high in protein, magnesium, and fiber (much higher than oatmeal), and has a low glycemic index. The GI of whole grain barley is only 22 (very low), and the cracked grain is only 50 (low for a grain).

Notice that dairy is 26% of the diet, primarily goat and sheep's milk. Of course, these are grass-fed animals, so the dairy is rich in omega-3 fatty acids and K2.

Nicoya Peninsula, Costa Rica

Grains	26 percent by weight
Dairy	24
Vegetables	14

Added sugars	11
Fruits	9
Legumes	7
Meat, poultry, fish	5
Eggs	2
Added fats	2

Here it looks like a bit of everything. Here we see animal products (dairy, meat, poultry, eggs, and fish) accounting for 31% of the diet. Grains are at 26%, and other vegetable products at 30%. Surprisingly, added sugar is rather high at 11%.

Seventh-Day Adventists

Vegetables	33 percent by weight
Fruits	27
Legumes and soy	12
Dairy	10
Grains	7
Meat and poultry	4
Added fats	2
Nuts and seeds	2
Fish	2
Eggs	1
Added sugar	1

Fresh fruits and vegetables come in at 81%. Interestingly, 16 per cent of the diet is animal products.

One Blue Zone in the US -- Loma Linda, California
I think the most interesting part of the Blue Zone study is the Seventh Day Adventists in Loma Linda, California.

I find them interesting because they are made up of a cross-section of people who live in the United States.

For small isolated cultures, a case can be made that the longevity is from their genes. Not so in Loma Linda. Let's look at this Blue Zone group more carefully.

Loma Linda University conducted several long-term studies trying to understand the correlation between lifestyle, diet, disease and mortality in the Seventh-day Adventists. These studies were conducted over a period of many years, beginning in 1960. The first study started with 22,940 participants (1960-1965). It had a 5-year follow-up and a 25-year follow-up. The study found that, compared to other Californians:

- Adventist men lived 6.2 years longer than non-Adventist men.
- Adventist women lived 3.7-years longer than non-Adventist women.
- Death rates from all cancers was 40% lower for Adventist men and 24% lower for Adventist women.
- Lung cancer was 79% lower.
- Colorectal cancer was 38% lower.
- Breast cancer was 15% lower.
- Coronary heart disease was 34% lower for Adventist men, and 2% lower for Adventist women.

In another study (1974-1988) the purpose was to find out exactly what was contributing to this difference. It involved approximately 34,000 participants.

This study found diet had a profound effect on both cancer and heart disease. In this study, Adventist men live 7.3 years longer and Adventist women live 4.4 years longer than other Californians.

If people just did these 5 things, they lived up to 10 years longer:

- Do not smoke.
- Eat a plant-based diet.
- Eat nuts several times per week.
- Get regular exercise.
- Maintain normal body weight.

In addition,

- Reducing consumption of red and white meat was associated with a decrease of colon cancer.
- Eating legumes was protective for colon cancer.
- Eating nuts several times a week reduces the risk of heart attack

by up to 50%.

- Eating whole-meal bread instead of white bread reduced non-fatal heart attack risk by 45%.
- Drinking 5 or more glasses of water per day may reduce heart disease by 50%.
- Men who had a high consumption of tomatoes reduced their risk of prostate cancer by 40%.
- Drinking soy milk more than once daily may reduce prostate cancer by 70%

Lower diseases in Adventists vs. the rest of America

- Death rates from all cancers were 40% lower for Adventist men and 24% lower for Adventist women
- Lung cancer 79% lower
- Colorectal cancer 38% lower
- Breast cancer 15% lower

There are other factors that may be contribution to their longevity.

- They grow their own food.
- They have a strong social network.

The other area that I think deserves more discussion is Okinawa.

According to the Pittsburgh Tribune, Japan (about the size of California) had 28,000 centenarians in 2005, where all of America had only 8,000. Wow!! Quite a difference! [104]

In Okinawa, people eat a large amount of sweet potatoes, up to 70 per cent of their diet.

The last 1% is made up of:

- nuts
- other potatoes
- seaweed
- sugars
- dairy
- eggs

- meat
- alcohol
- fish (very low considering it is an island)

In other words, this last 1% is what they are **not** eating.

What else do Okinawans do to achieve such longevity?

- They have a **support system**. When they are young, they are assigned to small groups that act as a support group for their entire lives.
- They practice *Hara hachi bu*. This is the practice of eating until your stomach is **80% full**. They eat smaller portions and eat more slowly. It can take up to 20 minutes for the stomach to tell the brain that it is full. Eating slowly lets this process happen.
- **They're happy.** Okinawans report being stress-free and have a positive outlook on life.
- **Eat very little in the late afternoon and evening**
- Eat mostly **plants**
- Eat **beans**
- Eat **meat rarely** and in small portions (3-4 oz) about 5 times per month, on average.
- Drink **alcohol moderately** and regularly (1-2 glasses per day)

Conclusion from Blue Zones

What does Dan Beuttner suggest we do to be more like the Blue Zones?

1. Eat whole real food, especially plants.

Many of the centenarians grow their own food. Rarely are they vegans or vegetarians (except the Seventh Day Adventists), but they eat only small amounts of animal products.

They primarily eat foods such as:

- vegetables
- fruit
- beans
- whole grains
- sweet potatoes

- nuts and seeds
- herbs
- eggs
- fish
- quality dairy products like grass-fed milk and cheese
- fermented products like yogurt and kefir

Most of them do eat meat, but rarely. They have meat on special occasions, and even then, it is a small part of the meal. I think it is important to note that these animal products are grass-fed, locally raised, free of hormones, antibiotics and pesticides, and wild caught. Therefore, they are much more nutritious than most meat found in the U.S.

2. Avoid Processed and Packaged Foods

The Blue Zone inhabitants eat locally grown real food. No chemicals, no pesticides, no artificial ingredients. They rarely add sweeteners to their food. For dessert they might eat something like cheese and fruit. There are no candy bars, sports drinks or sugary baked goods.

3. Get rid of unhealthy foods in your kitchen.

Go through your kitchen and get rid of all processed and packaged foods. That alone will make a huge difference in your health.

Only have real food in your kitchen. Americans are fat and unhealthy in part due to habit. It is much easier to eat a healthy diet if you only have healthy food around you.

Typically, Blue Zone inhabitants are slender throughout their lives. They don't have to think about dieting because all of their options are healthy.

4. Get into the habit of noticing exactly how full you are.

In Japan, the blue zones centenarians often practice the tradition of "hara hachi bu" which is eating until only 80 percent full.

5. Get a good night of sleep.

Blue Zoners typically get a full 8 hours of sleep. Sleep helps control hunger and other cravings

Inadequate sleep can take years off your life. Having trouble sleeping? Try exercising and eating a healthy diet.

6. Do some form of exercise every day

Make being active a part of your daily life. Most of being overweight is due to overeating and eating unhealthy foods. Although some calories are burned during exercise, there are many other reasons to exercise besides maintaining weight. Exercising keeps muscles working, and helps maintain flexibility and balance.

Rebuttal to the Blue Zones information:

The following rebuttal was taken from *The Carnivore Code* by Paul Saladino. [105] *Italics are my comments.*

The Blue Zones may have been selected for their plant-based diets

Saladino says that "there are other regions of the world that demonstrate similar degrees of longevity that were left out of the Blue Zones. Hong Kong has one of the highest life expectancies in the world (85 years) and is also the world's third largest consumer of beef per capita, with an average consumption of almost 1.5 pounds of total meat per day." [105]

In all fairness, the blue zones were not chosen for average life expectancy, but instead for which areas have the most people who live to be over 100. These are somewhat different groups.

Saladino gives several examples from research that show that a diet high in meat is actually correlated with living longer. He also says that "the epidemiology literature does not suggest a clear correlation between plant-based diets and longevity nor a detrimental effect of meat in the diet. In some cases, increased red meat is even associated with improved all-cause mortality."

Eating meat may increase Telomere length

Telomere length is one way to measure how we are aging. Longer telomeres are associated with longevity. Poor lifestyle choices can shorten telomeres. However, healthy lifestyle choices can actually lengthen telomeres. What kinds of things? Adequate sleep, exercise, moderate sunlight exposure, finding meaning in our lives, and a tight

-knit community.

What about food? "There is only one thing that is correlated with longer telomeres, and it's not plant foods. *It's red meat!*" [105]

The Blue Zoners may eat more meat than reported

According to Saladino, Dan Beuttner misrepresented the diets of all of the foreign Blue Zones. He says that these Blue Zones eat more meat and meat products (like cooking in animal fat) than Beuttner reports in his books. "Unfortunately, it seems that the central nature of the animal foods in the diets of Nicoyans, Sardinians, Okinawans, and Ikarians was ignored in the conceptualization of the Blue Zones." [105]

And then there is the Blue Zone in Southern California, the Seventh Day Adventists. He says that the Mormons see a similar increase in longevity, and they eat meat. Saladino suggests that it is not the diet, but instead healthy lifestyle choices such as not smoking, no alcohol, and living in a close community, that increases longevity.

My comments:

I know this is so confusing!! What should we believe? The Blue Zones books seem so convincing, and yet here is an excellent rebuttal. Which is true? Maybe the lesson here is to eat real food (no processed and packaged food), and if you eat meat, eat healthy meat (no hormones, antibiotics, and from animals that eat healthy food). How much meat to eat may vary from person to person. See what works for you. Keep in mind that the rebuttal was written by a carnivore. My opinion is that organic fruits and vegetables are good for our bodies and our microbiome.

By contrast, what do we eat in America?

As percentage of calories: *(Italics are mine)*

- 63% processed food (the fats are usually unhealthy seed oils, sugars, refined grains). *These are almost exclusively foods that have very little nutrition, and probably are made from plants that were sprayed with poison.*
- 25% animal food (meat, dairy, eggs, fish, seafood). *These are*

mostly animals that were raised with hormones, pesticides, antibiotics, and are fed GMO corn and soy (high in omega 6), and are therefore quite unhealthy.

- 12% plant food (vegetables, fruit, beans, nuts, seeds and whole grains). *These are primarily conventionally farmed with herbicides and pesticides. This is the healthiest category, but it still is contaminated with poison.* [106]

Given how we eat, it shouldn't be surprising that we are so unhealthy.

Other thoughts about aging

How long can we live?

The oldest documented people in the world are women.

- Jeanne Calment of France (1875-1997) lived to 122.
- Sarah Knauss of the United States (1880-1999) lived to 119.

The longest lifespan for a man is:

- Jiroeman Kimura of Japan (1887-2013) who lived to age 116. [107]

Usually, the oldest woman in the world, at any one time, lives to about 117, and the oldest men are about 111.

However, there seems to be a gene at play here, as this very old trait seems to run in families, and there does not seem to be an easy environmental explanation. Consequently, this information is not so useful for the rest of us who might hope to live to 115.

For people without that special gene, we can still live a long and healthy life by following the recommendations in this book. How long? **A normal life expectancy of good health for those of us who take good care of ourselves is about 90 or older, with some few making it past 100.**

If you are just starting healthier habits, do not despair! Our bodies want to be healthy. I think it is never too late to chart our course towards health.

Telomeres

I first heard about the importance of telomeres with regard to aging when I was in college, 50 years ago. This is not new information.

Telomeres are like the shoe lace tips on shoe laces. These tips are on the end of each DNA strand. I am sure you have seen pictures of your DNA. It looks sort of like an "X". So, there are 4 telomeres for each "X". Every time you make a new cell, and these DNA strands divide and duplicate, and your telomeres get slightly shorter. When the telomeres are completely gone, the cell dies. When enough cells die in this manner, then the person dies.

Most cells in your body are replaced every few months, some faster than others. For example, the cells on the lining of your small intestine are replaced every 2-5 days. Your skin epidermis cells are replaced every 10-39 days, your bones are replaced 10% per year, [108] and your brain and spinal cord you have for a lifetime (although new research says that we can grow new brain cells, at least in the hippocampus). [109]

I learned in college that poor nutrition speeds the loss of telomeres, whereas excellent nutrition can not only stop the deterioration of telomeres, but now we think that the right kind of food can actually add length to telomeres. Other things we can do to slow or reverse telomere length is to reduce stress, stop smoking, lose weight, and exercise more.

Building blocks of cells

In addition to the telomeres getting gradually shorter, **every time a cell divides, it is vital that there is adequate nutrition to build that new cell.**

Cells are very complicated. They have so many different parts that are needed to make them function properly. Do you remember learning about these in high school biology? See if you recognize some of these names:

There are **mitochondria**, the power plants of the cell.

The **nucleus** is where the DNA is kept. It is the cell "brain" of the cell and controls all of the other functions of the cell.

Ribosomes are where RNA is translated into protein.

The **endoplasmic reticulum** is the transport system for molecules.

The **lysosome** is the digestive system in the cell.

The **cell membrane** functions as a semi-permeable barrier. It controls what goes in and out of the cell.

The **cytoplasm** is the material, mostly water, inside the cell. Most of the parts of the cell are suspended in the cytoplasm.

Microtubules function in cell division and serve as a "temporary scaffolding" for other organelles.

Then there are **vacuoles, Golgi bodies, and chloroplasts**. [110]

It is vital to our health that we continuously eat the right kind of micronutrients to provide the building blocks to make all of the various parts of these cells.

It is possible that we may have no need for carbohydrates at all, in spite of the fact that most researchers say to eat primarily vegetables. [13]

Consequently, I think that if you are eating a healthy diet, even if that is primarily meat and fat, you may not have to worry about your fiber intake. However, everyone is different. See what works for you.

Personal note: I eat mostly non-starchy vegetables. I choose to believe that we do better with healthy gut bacteria (microbiome), and our microbiome needs a variety of fiber to eat. Maybe that is not true for everyone, but it works for me. In addition, we get a large range of nutrients from our vegetables. I once counted the number of different fruits and vegetables that I eat in a year, and it was about 75. That is a tiny range compared to primitive man, but it is a good range of the food easily available to us.

Are we just a victim of our genes?

Medical research has been focusing on genes as the cure for diseases for most of my lifetime. The belief has been that if we could only identify the specific gene that controls a certain disease, then we could control that disease. For some few diseases, this may be helpful, but it turns out that most diseases are a complex of many genes working together.

Let's look at different diseases and see if the theory that genes are causing diseases makes any sense. We are talking about nature vs. nurture. Do we come this way, or are we doing something to create our diseases? If we are causing the diseases, then we can change what we are doing and eliminate them. Inherited genes are stable over time. It takes a very long time for genes to change in a population. However, the environment can cause changes very rapidly. Let's see which one makes sense.

Diabetes. Over one third of the population is now diabetic or prediabetic

There are eight times as many diabetics now in the United States as there were in 1900.

Genes don't change that quickly. These changes are from the environment.

Heart Disease and Cancer. Heart disease and cancer are now the leading causes of death. In 2010 they accounted for 47% of all deaths, compared to 12% in 1900.

Again, genes don't change that quickly. These changes are from the environment.

Obesity. Over two-thirds (67.5%) of American adults are currently overweight or obese.

Obesity rates in children have tripled in 30 years.

One third of children are overweight or obese.

In spite of the fact that 70% of our tendency to be fat or thin is genes, we have seen a large change over a short time period. **That is not genes.** That is the 30% that we do have control over at work.

Autism. The clearest example is autism. Autism in 1975 was 1 in 5,000 in America. Now it is 1 in 38 (CDC). For easy numbers to understand, in 2013 it was 1 in 50, so it went from 1 in 5,000 in 1975, to 1 in 50 in 2013, or **100 times as many autistic children in only 38 years!** [111] These numbers vary somewhat, but are fairly similar in all Western countries.

That is not a genetic cause. Genes don't change that quickly. It has to be something we are doing to create so much autism in such a short amount of time.

I believe that the part that genes play is in determining which disease will show up.

For the most part, the cause for all of these "diseases of affluence" (see list below) is the environmental, not genetic. Why do different diseases show up? Genes may determine which disease you get, depending on what your genetic weak spot may be. In this way, genes play a part in choosing the disease, but the cause and the cure are both food and lifestyle choices.

Some people might be eating too much sugar, and maybe someone else might have a toxic mold situation. Perhaps another has been eating fish with too much mercury and has mercury poisoning. These are examples of environmental contributors to diseases.

I recommend that you and your family clean up your lives. Follow as many of the suggestions in this book that you are willing to do.

What percentage of these illnesses would go away if we ate healthy food?

Unhealthy eating habits can be an underlying cause of all of these physical issues. These are often called the "diseases of affluence" because, as a country becomes affluent, they change their eating habits and their customs, and these diseases start showing up in large numbers.

Exactly what are these "diseases of affluence"?

- Heart attacks
- Cancer
- Diabetes
- Alzheimer's
- Multiple sclerosis (MS)
- Auto-immune diseases
- Joint pain
- Irritability
- Bloating
- Autism
- Irregular sleep
- Hormone fluctuations
- Energy crashes
- Arthritis
- Asthma
- Digestive disorders, such as irritable bowel syndrome, acid reflux, and heartburn
- Fatigue and chronic fatigue
- Food allergies and sensitivities
- Headaches and migraines

- Parkinson's disease
- Depression
- Mood disorders such as depression and anxiety

This may not be a complete list.

Epigenetics and the "100 year effect"

There is also the **epigenetic factor**. This is the idea that genes are turned on or off, depending on our environment, including how we take care of ourselves. That means that even genes are not fixed, but rather very changeable in terms of their expression, depending on what we do.

We inherit our chromosomes from our parents. That doesn't change. The gene theory says that if you inherit a dominant gene, that gene will express itself. If you didn't get the gene, you won't have that trait. For example, if you have the gene for brown eyes, you will have brown eyes.

It is actually more complicated than that.

The egg that became me was made when my mother was a fetus inside my grandmother. According to Kent Thornburg, our genes are influenced by the nutrition of our ancestors through the process of **epigenetics.** He says that our grandmother's health and nutrition influenced what genes were turned on or off inside our mothers. If our grandmother's nutrition was poor, genes may have been turned down, like a dimmer switch on a light. Our mother's nutrition while we were a fetus influenced which genes got turned on or off. Our nutrition throughout our lives influenced which genes get turned on or off. Poor nutrition as a fetus or a child has an impact on how well we age, and what diseases we get. I am now 72 years old. The egg that made me was created in 1914 (when my mother was a fetus), so I am really a bit over 100 years old. This is known as the "100-year effect". [112]

Instead of blaming our mothers or grandmothers, let's instead address the fact that the American population has allowed the food industry to guide our food choices. If we want to be healthy, we need to take back that control, and start making better decisions about what we eat. [112]

Take away:

- The Blue Zones give us a great view into what some indigenous cultures eat to stay healthy and live long lives. Generally, they eat a variety of fresh organic vegetables, and a modest amount of meat. In addition to eating healthy food, they also engage in activities that support longevity, such as getting enough sleep and exercise, and participating in a community.
- Other factors that may influence longevity are telomere length and making sure you get enough nutrition every day to feed all of your cells and build new ones.

Chapter 7

Preventing and Reversing Diseases

Insulin sensitivity is going to determine, for the most part, how long you are going to live and how healthy you are going to be. It determines the rate of aging more so than anything else we know right now.

--Ron Rosedale, M.D. [40]

Causes of most chronic diseases

When you don't take care of your body, many things go wrong. The words "inflammation", "metabolic disorder", "metabolic syndrome", "mitochondrial disfunction", "insulin resistance", or "insulin sensitivity" are all ways to measure illness. These are the underlying issues in almost all chronic illnesses. Let's start with inflammation because that is one we all can easily understand.

Inflammation

Inflammation is the body's attempt to heal itself.
There are 2 types of inflammation: acute and chronic.

Acute inflammation is what happens when you hit your thumb with a hammer. It gets red and swollen, but then begins to heal.

Chronic inflammation may go on for many months or years. An example of chronic inflammation is arthritis.

What happens during inflammation?

- Your body releases more cortisol. This makes the heart work harder. It also uses magnesium, so, over time, we develop a shortage of magnesium. This leads to increased heart palpitation, and your arteries become hardened.
- Your body also releases adrenalin.
- Your blood vessels tighten.

Chronic inflammation creates damage rather than benefit.

What causes chronic inflammation? Lifestyle. It's all under your control. Instead of saying, "I have arthritis, or a heart condition," instead say, "I have a symptom that tells me that I have inflammation in my body. And then ask, "How could I lower my inflammation?"

There are so many health conditions that have exploded in prevalence just in my lifetime. I was not aware of peanut allergies or autism as a child. They were very rare conditions. Now so many diseases are commonplace. Why? All lifestyle. When I was a child almost all kids were lean and healthy. We played outside all afternoon, including in the dirt. We didn't worry much about bacteria.

Now these diseases are rampant:

- Peanut allergy, or all types of allergies
- Autism
- Obesity
- Diabetes
- Leaky gut
- Heart conditions in younger people
- Cancers – all ages, instead of being a disease of the elderly

These seem to be the primary contributing factors to inflammation:

- Food
- Stress (maybe a big stressor like a divorce)

- Sleep (not enough, or interrupted sleep)
- Mental attitude (anxiety, depression)
- Lack of positive connections with others
- Lack of exercise

Be aware of your inflammation. How inflamed are you?

To avoid inflammation, you should be able to answer a resounding "yes" to all of these questions:

- Are you eating food with adequate nutrition?
- Do you exercise at least 30 minutes per day?
- Is your BMI in the normal range?
- Do you drink adequate healthy water with no fluoride or chlorine, and natural minerals?
- Do you avoid foods that spike your blood sugar?
- Are you eating primarily non-starchy vegetables?
- Are you eating enough healthy fats?
- Do you get at least 7 hours of sleep, without taking medication?
- Do you have fulfilling relationships?
- Do you manage your stress well?
- Do you have healthy teeth and gums?

Fatty liver disease

Robert Lustig is a researcher at UCSF where he works with obese children and adults. **His conclusions are that fatty liver disease is the driver of chronic diseases.** What causes fatty liver disease? Four foods. These are all metabolized similarly in the liver:

- **Fructose.** Sugar is half fructose and half glucose. Fructose has become a major cause of fatty liver disease.
- **Alcohol.** Until recently this was the primary cause of fatty liver.
- **Trans fats.** These have mostly been eliminated.
- **Branch chain amino acids.** The unhealthy versions are a problem, such as beef from feed lots.

Before 1980, fatty liver disease was mainly found in alcoholics. Non-alcoholic fatty liver disease hadn't even been identified. Now it is the leading cause of liver transplants in women. [29]

Metabolic syndrome

Metabolic syndrome is defined as having at least 3 of the following 5 conditions: [113]

- **Abdominal obesity:** as measured by a waist circumference of over 40 inches for men and over 35 inches for women.
- **Low HDL:** less than 40 mg/dl for men and less than 50 mg/dl for women, or taking medication.
- **High blood pressure:** over 130 mmHg systolic (the top number) or over 85 mmHg diastolic (the bottom number), or taking medication.
- **High triglycerides:** over 150 mg/dl, or taking medication.
- **Fasting blood glucose:** greater than 100 mg/dl, or taking medication.

Almost one third of the adult population of North America qualifies as having metabolic syndrome. **Having these characteristics increases the risk of having heart disease by almost 300%. In fact, the top 3 diseases (heart disease, cancer, and diabetes), are all related to metabolic syndrome. [77]**

Note that LDL is not part of this syndrome.

All of these symptoms have a common cause: too much insulin, or hyperinsulinemia. [114]

Interestingly, these tend to have a progression of appearing in the body. The first to appear is weight gain, even as little as a few pounds. This is followed by low HDL. Then high blood pressure, fatty liver and high triglycerides are next to appear. The last to appear is high blood glucose. At this point, the person is probably diagnosed with type 2 diabetes. [77]

Dr. Jason Fung suggests that all of these symptoms are really solutions to a problem. What is the problem? Too much sugar. "We need to get rid of the sugar and lower insulin." He goes on to say, **"When we treat the root cause, then type 2 diabetes, and indeed the entire metabolic syndrome, is a completely reversible disease"** [77]

What are some of the symptoms of poor metabolic health?

- Abdominal obesity

- Skin tags
- Dark areas around neck and armpits
- Erectile dysfunction
- Fungal infections, such as thrush
- Prominent sock marks (an indentation that stays – this could indicate heart failure) [87]

In summary, "inflammation", "metabolic disorder", "metabolic syndrome", "mitochondrial disfunction", "insulin resistance", or "insulin sensitivity" are the underlying factors in almost all chronic diseases. The good news is that these conditions are primarily controlled by food and lifestyle choices, so they are largely under our control.

Let's look at some of these diseases in more detail.

Which diseases can be prevented or reversed with food and lifestyle choices

---

Entire books have been written on each disease. I am going to cover just a few diseases to show that reversing diseases might be accomplished with diet and lifestyle changes. I am not giving medical advice. Talk to your health care professional about your own individual care. However, if your doctor says that chronic diseases cannot be reversed with diet and lifestyle changes, you might consider finding a new doctor.

Covid-19

As I am writing this book, Covid-19 is the illness getting most of the attention. Although it is not a chronic disease, it is largely preventable with food and lifestyle changes.

The *Journal of the American Medical Association* found:

- 94% of those who have been hospitalized with Covid had a pre-existing condition.
- 88% had 2 or more pre-existing conditions.
- Obesity is the number one pre-existing condition -- by far.

- Next is hypertension and diabetes. [115]

Covid is now part of the world. There is a lethal virus out there. You can make yourself healthy enough that it should not be an issue for you, or you can have one or more of the pre-existing conditions and possibly get very sick and even die. Even if you are slender and look healthy, you may still have chronically high insulin levels, which may put you into the danger zone.

At some point, we need to address why some people get so sick with it, and what we can do about it.

"Eat less, exercise more" does not work. Eating the "standard American diet" does not work. It is time to start telling the truth about what does work, and give people the tools they can use to make themselves healthier. [115]

In case you are unsure what these tools are, read the section on what the government recommendation *should* be, or read the section on boosting your immune system.

Heart attacks and strokes

Atherosclerosis and heart disease were virtually unknown
until we invented processed carbohydrates. They create metabolic
syndrome. Metabolic syndrome sets the scene in the body for
perpetual inflammation.
In that situation any injury to the endothelium cannot be healed.
--Natasha Campbell-McBride [44]

Heart disease is the number one killer in the Western world. One third of all deaths in developed countries are from coronary heart disease (CHD). The death rate from CHD reached its peak in the 1950's, and is less now, due to new medical procedures, such as drugs, bypass surgery, balloon angioplasty, and heart transplants.

About one half of the people who have a heart attack die in the first 2-3 hours. For many of these, the first symptom of heart disease is death. [44]

However, CHD is now reaching epidemic proportions, especially in the developing countries. [116]

Yet, before 1900, CHD was very rare. What has changed since 1900?

If we can figure out what has changed, we will know the cause of CHD.

Conventional medicine seems to *not know* how to prevent or cure CHD. They have identified "risk factors" such as "smoking, obesity, diabetes, high blood pressure, physical inactivity, male gender, family history of arterial disease, stress, and an anxious and aggressive personality". [44] These are contributors to heart disease.

However, the "risk factors" that we hear the most about are **cholesterol and fats. These are not contributors to heart disease.**

Lowering cholesterol and reducing fat are big money-makers. Cholesterol-lowering medications are the biggest money-making drugs in the world. The food industry has made a fortune selling "low fat" foods.

Let's look at what really causes heart disease:

Q: When does heart disease begin?

A: Heart disease is a progressive illness. It begins earlier than you might think. It actually begins for everyone as a child. By the time symptoms appear, it is in the advanced stages. There is no test to determine how bad it is until very late in the process.

Q: How do we know it begins so early?
A: Autopsies. After death we can look at the artery walls and assess the damage. In one study, over 3,000 young people who had died in accidents or as a result of suicides were studied. They were between 14 and 35 years old. It was found that 20-25% of them had a major lesion in the coronary arteries.

Even teenagers may have the beginnings of coronary atherosclerosis. Tuzcu et al, found that about 20% of teenagers had measurable coronary atherosclerosis in hearts available for transplant. [117]

Q: What exactly happens to the heart to create coronary atherosclerosis?
The following is a simplified version of the process. For a more detailed version, I suggest reading: *When does heart disease begin (and what that tells us about prevention)?* By Peter Attia, M.D. found online at peterattiamd.com, or read *Reverse Heart Disease Now* by Sinatra and Roberts. [117]

A: **We are born with smooth artery walls with a single layer of cells protecting the outside of the wall**. Cholesterol is a fat that is carried around in your blood. Because cholesterol is a fat, it needs to be carried through your blood (which is mostly water) because fat and water don't mix. These "carriers" are like little boats that take your cholesterol to the cells in your body. These "boats" are called LDL (low density lipoproteins) and HDL (high density lipoproteins).

These "boats" carry not just cholesterol, but also triglycerides, and phospholipids. There are two kinds of LDL. There are the very small LDL (VLDL) and the larger, fluffy LDL particles.

Cholesterol is vital to our existence and has a very important function in every cell of our bodies. All tissues make cholesterol, but some don't make enough, so our blood needs to bring them more.

Sometimes these cholesterol "boats" (LDL particles), with their cholesterol passenger, pass through the artery lining and get stuck just outside the artery wall. It is thought that these are mostly the small LDL particles, not the large fluffy ones. There they become oxidized. Think of oxidizing like iron rusting. Oxidation is unhealthy. As more and more of these LDL particles accumulate, they irritate the lining of the artery. Up to this point, the inner wall still looks smooth and flows well. It is just the area outside the artery wall that is getting irritated. This process starts in the first decade of life.

As more and more oxidized LDL accumulates outside of the artery wall, eventually the edges bulge into the artery and sometimes break into the artery itself. Cholesterol plaque comes along to seal the injury inside the artery wall. Over time, layers of plaque build up. This is when we begin to see the disease. We can measure the plaque buildup inside the artery. **Plaque is traditionally blamed for the disease, but it is actually just acting as band aid to cover the damaged artery.** Plaque on the inside of the artery is not the enemy. It is a symptom of the amount of cholesterol that has broken through the artery wall.

The disease has been progressing for many years by the time plaque appears in the artery wall.

Eventually, the plaque on the inside of the artery wall gets so thick that part of it breaks off, travels down the artery and creates a clog, or the thickness of the plaque gets to the point that the artery is completely clogged.

This is a heart attack if it is in the heart, or a stroke if it is in the brain. This clogging action can happen anywhere in our bodies, but if it happens in our heart or brain, it can be fatal.

How old are we when cardiac events, such as a heart attack, begin? Women are about 10-20 years behind men in having cardiac events. About twice as many men as women have heart attacks at age 45-54. About 24% of all events happen for men in age 45-54. For women, about 13% of all events occur then. [118]

Half of all cardiac events occur before age 65 for men, and one third of all events occur for women by age 65. Let that sink in. These are young people already having cardiac events.

Doctors and patients typically don't start taking cardiac prevention seriously until about age 60. By the age of 60, 100% of people have some signs of atherosclerosis. [119] However, because there are so many more 45 to 64-year-olds in the population, the perception is that cardiac events are rare at that age.

By age 85-94, not many people are still alive, so the percent of death by heart attack increases dramatically.

How can we prevent or at least slow this progression? Let's go back to what starts the problem: the LDL "boat" with its cholesterol passenger breaking through the artery wall and going where they should not be.

So, the question really is: **Why do the artery walls allow the LDL particles to go through?** The single layer of cells lining the artery wall is supposed to be a protective barrier. However, **inflammation damages the artery walls and allows breaks to occur, letting the LDL particles through into areas where they don't belong.**

What causes inflammation? Primarily what we eat, but also other lifestyle choices. Foods that cause inflammation are **anything that spikes blood sugar (like sugar and flour) combined with processed vegetable oils. These are the enemy of artery wall health.**

One of the standard medical views is that there are too many LDL particles. When there are too many, some break through the artery wall. (Attia) Not everyone agrees with this. So, if this is the case, the job of the doctor is to reduce the number of LDL particles. I don't happen to agree with this view, given the other research I have read.

Some say that only the small LDL particles (VLDL) break through the artery lining. The large fluffy LDL particles are not a problem. We can measure these. If your LDL is high, but your VLDL is low, then perhaps the high total LDL is not a problem. [40]

In addition, some cultures do not show this progression of heart

damage. Consequently, progressive heart disease is not an inevitable part of the human aging, but rather a result of eating the Western diet.

Benjamin Bikman, Ph.D.

Benjamin Bikman, Ph.D. says "insulin resistance and cardiovascular disorders are almost inseparable." [115]

In addition, if there is high blood pressure over a prolonged period of time, this leads to heart failure. Almost all people with hypertension are insulin resistant. He says that "insulin resistance and high insulin levels directly cause high blood pressure."

He concludes by saying, "Though we often blame other factors, there is no single variable more relevant to heart disease than insulin resistance. Any successful efforts to reduce our high risk of heart disease must address it. When we acknowledge the central role of insulin resistance, we start resolving the fundamental causes, rather than the symptoms (which is all medications can do.) As much as worldwide efforts to stem heart disease have tried, the longer we overlook insulin resistance, the worse the problem will get." [115]

Dwight Lundell, M.D.

Dwight Lundell, M.D., was a heart surgeon who performed over 5,000 coronary bypass surgeries. Over the years, he began to be a little troubled. In spite of the medical profession saying that high cholesterol caused heart disease, **he noticed that most of his patients had normal cholesterol levels.** Even if they came back 10 years later for another heart operation, they still had normal cholesterol. So why was the medical community saying that heart disease was caused by high cholesterol? He could see that high cholesterol was not causing heart disease in his patients.

He studied the medical research literature. He found a study published in 2009 which reviewed 136,000 patients admitted to the hospital with heart attacks. **Seventy per cent of these heart attack patients had normal cholesterol.** It became clear to him that high cholesterol was not the cause of heart attacks, in spite of the fact that the American Heart Association said it was.

So, what was causing heart disease?

From looking at so many hearts on the operating table, he made the observation that there was "redness and swelling around the plaque area." Redness and swelling are signs of **inflammation.** Could that be what is causing heart disease?

What causes inflammation? He believed it to be sugar and other carbohydrates that spike blood sugar.

Why did he suspect high blood sugar? The US dietary guidelines came out in 1977 which told us to stop eating saturated fats, and instead eat 60-70% of our calories as carbohydrates. That is when the explosion of obesity and diabetes began. Saturated fats do raise LDL cholesterol, but if LDL cholesterol does not cause heart attacks, then "elimination of saturated fats makes no sense." [59]

Near the end of his surgical career, he suggested to the hospital that they address the true causes of heart disease, namely diet. The hospital did not support this idea. He believed that they rejected his ideas because addressing the cause of heart disease was a "threat to their revenue stream." [59] In other words, they had no interest in keeping people healthy. They wanted to continue sending huge bills to the insurance companies for heart surgeries.

Soon after that he closed his surgical practice and opened a clinic that focused on low-carbohydrate nutrition. He wanted to find out if his ideas were correct. Yes! He was right. He was very successful in reversing not only heart disease, but diabetes as well.

He wrote a book and gave many speeches to try to get the word out.

How did the medical community respond? Four years after he retired, the Arizona Medical Board took away his medical license.

The Vegan Solution to Heart Issues

Caldwell Esselstyn, Jr. M.D.

I think one of the most impressive researchers on heart disease is Caldwell Esselstyn, Jr. M.D. He wrote a book *Prevent and Reverse Heart Disease*. [30] In this book he talks about his experiences as a heart surgeon. He realized that heart surgery was only dealing with the symptoms of heart disease, but was doing nothing for the underlying cause of the disease. He decided to try something. He took 24 people who were extremely ill and started them on a very strict program of eating. The popular movie, *Forks Over Knives*, summarizes his research.

Between them they had had 49 cardiovascular events, including:

- 7 cases of bypass surgery
- 4 heart attacks
- 3 strokes
- 2 angioplasty procedures
- 15 cases of increased angina
- 13 cases of measurable disease progression
- 2 worsening stress tests

Most of them were very desperate. Many of them were heading towards imminent death.

They had to strictly follow his program. The rules were simple. Maybe not easy to follow, but simple. He only included people who were very motivated to follow the plan. Out of the 24 who began, 18 people stuck with his program through the first year.

His rules:

- Do not eat meat or fish or any animal products (no eggs, no milk, no cheese)
- No oil of any kind
- Only whole grains
- Do not drink fruit juice (whole fruit is OK)
- No nuts or avocados or coconut products (because of the oil)
- No salt

What does that leave?

The huge range of vegetables, fruits, and whole grains.

After 12 years, Dr. Esselstyn reports:
"Among the fully compliant patients, during the twelve-year study, there was not one further clinical episode of worsening coronary artery disease."

In contrast, for the 6 who dropped out of the program, the illness progressed.

Dr. Esselstyne's diet has very impressively prevented and reversed heart disease for many people.

However, these are the downsides with this diet as I see it.

With a vegan diet, it is important to take supplements. Vitamin B12 is essential. Dr. Esselstyn also recommends Vitamin D3, and Omega-3 fatty acids.

I believe we are meant to eat real food, not supplements. Following this thinking, we are probably meant to eat some animal products to get adequate B12.

Also, he says that people do not need to pay attention to the amount that is eaten. No more counting calories. I believe that many people still need to watch how much they eat. However, his diet has no fat, no sugar, and no processed foods, so maybe it is easier to stay slim on his diet.

He says not to worry about how much protein you are consuming. He says there is plenty of protein in his diet. He could be right. His patients seem to be doing fine by following his program. However, I have some concerns about this.

Dr. Esselstyne recommends a low-fat, plant-based diet. Using this program, he was very successful in reversing severe heart disease in his patients. Interestingly, what Dr. Esselstyne's program and the high-fat programs have in common is eliminating all processed foods.

In support of his ideas, there is the Blue Zone of Okinawa where people eat 97% vegetables, almost no animal protein or fat, and they are healthy and live long lives. [102]

Bottom line: Dr. Esselstein successfully stopped the progression and even reversed the damage to cardiac patients by changing their diets to low-fat, plant-based food.

High fat, low carb diets successfully prevent heart disease for most people, and low-fat, plant-based diets are also successful.

What do these diets have in common? Eating real food. No processed or packaged food. Maybe that is the change that is needed to prevent and reverse heart disease.

Cancer

In recent years, scientists have come to realize that it's not genetic mutations that cause cancer. We now know that mitochondrial damage happens first. . . When you remove processed foods, sugar, grains, and high-net-carb fuels from your diet, you essentially stress cancer cells by depriving them of their preferred metabolic fuel.

Dr. Joseph Mercola [14]

Some cancer facts

- Cancer is the second leading cause of death (heart disease is number one).
- Cancer can affect any organ.
- Breast cancer is the most common cancer in women.
- Prostate cancer is the most common cancer in men.
- Lung cancer is the deadliest.
- In spite of spending $160 billion each year in the US on cancer research, more and more people are dying of cancer each year. [115]

As Jason Fung, M.D. points out in *"The Cancer Code"*, "From 1969 to 2014, total deaths in the United States from heart disease dropped approximately 17 percent despite the increasing population. But cancer? During that sometime period, deaths from cancer rose a chilling *84 percent."* [23]

Are cancer drugs working? According to Jason Fung, "From 1990 to 2002, 71 new drug approvals were granted for 45 new drugs. Of those, only 12 medications were proven to save lives, and most extended life by only a few weeks or months." [23] That does not look very impressive to me.

What causes cancer?

Smoking is the leading cause of cancer, roughly responsible for 35% of cancer deaths, primarily from lung cancer.

The second factor in controlling cancer is diet/nutrition, which is responsible for about 30% of all cancers. [120]

According to Jason Fung, genes are, at most, responsible for 30% of all cancers. [23]

What about diet/nutrition can improve cancer risk?

- Most cancer cells burn only glucose. They cannot burn ketones.
- Most cells in our bodies can burn either glucose or ketones.
- Our cells run just fine, maybe even better, on just ketones.
- So, to kill cancer, eliminate glucose and run our bodies on

ketones.

- How? Eliminate or greatly reduce refined carbohydrates.
- Or eat mostly fat.
- Eat a moderate amount of protein (our bodies make protein into glucose if we eat too much protein).
- **So, starve the cancer by lowering glucose.** [23]

In 1924, Dr. Otto Warburg discovered that cancer cells burn glucose, and can't burn fat, for which he won the Nobel Prize in 1931. This is known as the Warburg effect.

Dr. Peter Pedersen from Johns Hopkins added that the cancer cells have a very low number of healthy mitochondria.

Dr. Thomas N. Seyfried, who wrote *Cancer as a Metabolic Disease* in 2012, explains that there are some cancers that do not have a genetic mutation. Instead, they damage the mitochondria, producing the Warburg effect. Read *Fat for Fuel* for a more thorough discussion. [14]

Insulin causes cancer cells to grow.

- People with hyperinsulinemia (excess insulin) have roughly double the likelihood of dying from cancer. [121]
- Researchers found that controlling insulin resistance helped control breast cancer. [122]
- Women with the highest fasting insulin levels are those with the worst breast cancer outcomes. [115] [123]

Low cholesterol may be linked to cancer:

- People with low cholesterol levels are prone to cancer. [124]
- If cholesterol is artificially lowered with a statin drug, the results can be increased risk of cancer, breast cancer in particular.

Other things that may help

Intermittent fasting for more than 13 hours per day may help prevent breast cancer recurrence. [125]

Drinking green tea may help delay the age of onset of cancer by 7.3 years. [126]

The rate of cancer depends more on your environment than your genes.

In twin studies, the increased risk of cancer in fraternal twins (similar to siblings) was only 5%. Even in identical twins (same genes), it was only 14%. [127] There clearly is a genetic component to cancer, but it is much lower than we are led to believe.

The cancer experience of the Canadian Inuit (Eskimos) is similar to other native populations. Cancer seems to have been essentially nonexistent in 1923, [128] and in 1949, a report found only fourteen cases of cancer in a ten-year period. [129]

After WWII many Inuit were forced out of their traditional lands, and began moving to larger urban areas. They abandoned their traditional diet of primarily fish and sea mammals (low in carbohydrates and vegetables and high in protein and fat) and began eating foods containing refined grains and sugars. In the 1950's the age-adjusted rate of cancer more than doubled.

The types of cancers also changed. The Inuit tended to have cancers caused by the Epstein-Barr virus, typically found in the nose and throat. Typical cancers in the white population, then and now, were lung, breast, and colon cancers. From 1950-1997, the rate of the Inuit traditional cancers did not increase, whereas the cancers associated with the white population rose from approximately 23 to 88 per 100,000 person years. [130]

Genes do not change that quickly. It was the change in food/environment that led to the increase in cancers. [23]

What happens when people migrate?

Are cancer rates similar to their country of origin (genes control cancer) or like their new country (environment controls cancer).

The rate of breast cancer in the United States is two to four times higher than in China or Japan. What happens when a Japanese or Chinese woman moves to the United States? The rate of breast cancer goes up. Within a few generations, the rate of breast cancer in Japanese and Chinese women who move to San Francisco approximates that of white women living in San Francisco (2 to 4 times higher than in Japan and China).

The rate of cancer is highly dependent on the environment – primarily diet and lifestyle. [23]

The same is found for Japanese men who move to Hawaii. After living in Hawaii, their rate of prostate cancer is seven times that of Japanese men who live in Osaka, Japan. Again, cancer increases so that the rate of cancer is similar to the new environment, indication that environment, not genes, are controlling these cancers.

Does the rate of any cancer decrease when Japanese men migrate to Hawaii? Yes, the rate for stomach cancer decreases after Japanese men move to Hawaii. The stomach cancer rate of Japanese men who live in Japan is 5 times that of Japanese men who move to Hawaii. [131] Again, the environment seems to control the rate of cancer, not genes.

Clearly, the environment is responsible for these changes in cancer rate, not genes.

In summary, genes are not the primary factor in whether or not we will get cancer. At most, genes contribute 30 percent of the risk factor for cancer. It is diet and lifestyle that are the primary contributors to cancer risk. That is good news. We have control over these.

The best way to prevent cancer is to not smoke, to limit all foods that increase insulin, to keep your weight under control, and to avoid type 2 diabetes.

Diabetes

Diabetes is the inevitable result of converting from a traditional diet to a modern one, as observed in Pima Indians, the Aboriginal people of Australia, and the tribes of the Amazon rain forest. All of these populations experienced virtually no obesity or diabetes on their traditional diet but displayed epidemic levels of obesity and diabetes within just a few years of being introduced to modern foods.
--William Davis, M.D. [85]

Is diabetes genetic?
Type I diabetes is genetic, and usually begins before age 40
Type 2 diabetes is primarily a lifestyle disease

Doctors who have success in reversing diabetes – what are they doing?
Dr. Jason Fung, an expert in curing diabetes through lifestyle, recommends the following: [77]

- **Avoid fructose**
- **Reduce refined carbohydrates**
- **Enjoy natural fats**
- **Eat real food**
- **Try intermittent fasting**

Let's look at these in more detail.

If diabetes is caused by having too much sugar in the blood and too much sugar in the cells, then the solution is to **reduce sugar**, fructose in particular (by changing what you eat), and allow the body to burn up the sugars that are already there (by not eating so often).

"The prevalence of diabetes climbs 1.1% for every extra 150 sugar calories per person per day." [77] [132]

Eating too much fructose causes fatty liver, and this leads directly to insulin resistance. Having a steady flow of glucose in the blood (eating throughout the day) leads to a steady high level of insulin. A steady high level of insulin is what leads to insulin resistance. Insulin resistance is the cause of diabetes.

Refined carbohydrates spike blood sugar and send a rush of glucose into the blood. However, sugar seems to be a much more potent toxin as far as diabetes is concerned. For example, the Chinese diet has traditionally been based on eating white rice (glucose), and yet they had very little obesity or type 2 diabetes until they began eating more sugar (half glucose and half fructose). As they added sugar to their diet, type 2 diabetes began to climb. **It seems that the fructose is the primary toxin, and is much more dangerous than glucose.**

Healthy fats, such as avocados, olive oil, and grass-fed beef, **do not increase blood sugar**, and help slow the release of glucose into the blood. However, remember that heavily processed seed and bean oils such as soybean, canola, and Crisco, are toxic.

Eating real food means **avoiding all of the processed foods** that are damaging our bodies.

Intermittent fasting can be limiting the number of hours we eat each day (fasting for 12-16 hours per day), or doing a water-only fast for a few days, or limiting calories a few days a week. In extreme cases, perhaps the most effective thing to start with is to not eat anything.

Let's explore this further.

Fasting to cure diabetes

Dr. Jason Fung is not only an expert on diabetes but also on fasting. He has written *The Diabetes Code* [77] and *The Complete Guide To Fasting.* [16]

Jason Fung, M.D., in an interview with Peter Attia, M.D., talks about how he deals with severe diabetics. He says that fasting is a potent antidote to obesity, insulin resistance, type 2 diabetes, and the many symptoms of metabolic illness. He tells his patients "Only eat between this hour and this hour, and don't eat anything that came in a box. . . to me, that is practical, useful advice." [133]

He says that people currently are eating about 15 hours a day. That is almost continuously eating during their waking hours. He says that it is much healthier to eat for only about 8 hours a day. He sees a lot of people who benefit from this one intervention alone. He points out it is so much easier to restrict eating to a certain time rather than counting carbs.

Dr. Peter Attia finds that some patients benefit from an eating window of 16/8 (eating for only 8 hours), but that others do not respond to this. Some people have to push it to as much as 22/2 to see a benefit (eating for only 2 hours per day). However, he says that there is no substitute for water fasting for 3 to 7 days, or restricting calories for 3 to 7 days (20-40% of normal calories).

What does Dr. Fung do if he sees a person with advanced diabetes? **He had a patient in his 40's who had a non-healing diabetic foot ulcer for about a year. This patient was on the verge of getting his foot amputated.** The diabetes was causing his foot ulcer. In order to heal the foot ulcer, he had to get his diabetes under control. **Dr. Fung started him on a week of fasting, then followed with fasting for 36 hours per week. The ulcer healed within 3 weeks. Within a few months, he was no longer diabetic. Even a few years later, he was no longer diabetic.**

Dr. Attia pointed out that if you get to the point of needing an amputation, the 5-year mortality rate is extremely high. The chances are that you won't live much longer.

Peter Attia does not start with a week of fasting because most people who are not used to fasting will be quite ill if they do not ease into fasting. However, Jason Fung deals with much sicker people. Sometimes they do not have the luxury of starting slowly.

Jason Fung offers fasting to everybody. He says that about 50% of people won't do it, not for any period of time, not even for

167

small amounts of time like 5 hours. **It is the psychological part that is difficult, not the physical part**. It's not fun, but it's not that difficult to actually do it. However, a supportive environment is very important. Other doctors, and friends and family, can make a huge impact on the success or failure of fasting.

Note: Jason Fung emphasizes that we are all different. He says most people do well on low carb diets, but some people do not do well. [134]

By contrast, what does the medical profession recommend for diabetics?

Kaiser Permanente follows the MyPlate recommendations of the U.S. government. Let's look at what is on their website. *Italics are mine.*

- "Half the plate is non-starchy vegetables. This is about the size of your closed fist, although you can go back for seconds on these foods. Examples are broccoli, green beans, carrots, mushrooms, tomatoes, cauliflower, spinach, peppers, and salad greens. "

Most high-fat and low-fat researchers seem to agree that most of what you eat should be fresh non-starchy vegetables. The usual recommendation is up to 80% of foods by volume. Kaiser recommends eating vegetables the size of your fist. This is their one excellent recommendation. However, it is not nearly enough. For example, Dr. Terry Wahls recommends 9 cups of vegetables per day.

- "One-fourth of the plate is a bread, starch, or grain. This is about the size of half a closed fist. Examples are bread, rolls, rice, crackers, cooked grains, cereal, tortillas, and starchy vegetables like potatoes, corn, winter squash, beans, peas, and lentils."

Bread, starch, or grains are acceptable to some researchers, but unacceptable to many. Grains spike blood sugar much like sugar does. Diabetics, especially, should avoid this. For diabetics anything made with grain should be eliminated, especially if sugar is also part of the diet. (I am not giving medical advice, just my opinion.)

- One-fourth is lean protein. This is about the size of a deck of cards. Examples are beef, chicken, turkey, pork, fish, tofu, and eggs. (For the plate format, beans should be counted as a starch, not as a protein.)

Protein is good, but Kaiser is very anti-fat, especially saturated fats. There are many researchers who recommend that we eat up to 80 % of our diet as healthy fats, including saturated fats, as measured in calories.

- Add a small piece of fruit. A small piece of fresh fruit is about the size of a tennis ball. Or choose ½ cup of frozen, cooked, or canned fruit. You could also have a small handful of dried fruit or ½ cup (4 ounces) of 100% fruit juice.

Fresh fruit is good. Frozen fruit is fine. Canned fruit has very little nutrition. Dried fruit has too much concentrated sugar. Fruit juice spikes blood sugar. It is not recommended because it has no fiber to slow down the sugar rush.

- Enjoy a cup (8 ounces) of low-fat or fat-free milk. If you don't drink milk, you could substitute with 6 ounces of no-sugar-added yogurt, another serving of fruit, or a small dinner roll.

Again, Kaiser is anti-fat. For the high-fat, low-carb researchers, if milk is recommended, they suggest whole-fat milk, just the way it comes from the cow (see discussion of milk in the ancestor section). Milk has lactose, a sugar. Casein is a protein in milk that many people have trouble digesting. Seventy-five per cent of the world has a problem digesting milk. The healthiest part is the fat. Yogurt with no added sugar is good. A dinner roll has calories but virtually no nutrition, and spikes blood sugar. It should therefore be avoided, especially for diabetics.

The belief in the medical profession is that diabetes is incurable. It can only be managed. Once someone is insulin resistant, they need ever-more-increasing amounts of insulin to survive, leading eventually to death.

In spite of what the medical profession is currently recommending, research shows that diabetes is largely curable through changes in food and lifestyle. [77]

Multiple Sclerosis

Dr. Terry Wahls

She was able to reverse Multiple Sclerosis (MS) with diet and lifestyle changes.

Dr. Terry Wahls is a physician who had debilitating MS and eliminated her symptoms herself through diet and lifestyle.

She was relatively young when she was first diagnosed with Multiple Sclerosis in 2000. MS is an autoimmune disease that damages the brain and spinal cord. It is the most common cause of early disability in the US. She began taking drugs which cost almost a thousand dollars a month. According to Dr. Wahls, some of the side-effects of MS drugs are: body aches, depression, mouth sores, heart problems, a higher risk of life-threatening infections, and even death. Over a period of 6 years, her MS gradually progressed until she was wheelchair-bound. She was so weak and easily fatigued that she eventually needed to use a recumbent wheelchair. She could not sit up in a regular wheelchair.

She had been treating the MS very aggressively with state-of-the-art medical care. She went to the Cleveland Clinic because it was one of the top medical facilities in the US for treating MS. She was an internist who believed in the medical system, such as using the latest drugs. In spite of that, her disease steadily progressed.

In 2002, she discovered *The Paleo Diet* by Loren Cordain, Ph.D. [135] The paleo diet consists of food that we believe we ate back when we were hunter/gatherers. This is meat, fruit, and vegetables. No grains, beans, or dairy.

Terry Wahls had been a vegetarian for the previous 20 years. She was eating what seemed like an extremely healthy diet.

As a vegetarian for 20 years, she ate:

- wheat bread
- beans
- rice
- a variety of fruits and vegetables

She did not eat:

- processed food

- white flour
- sugar

This diet looks really healthy, doesn't it? And yet, she was getting sicker and sicker!

It was difficult for her to consider eating meat, but the research persuaded her to give it a try. Note: she had not been taking a vitamin B12 supplement, which is recommended for vegans.

She added meat to her diet, and eliminated grains, dairy, and legumes. Her decline slowed, but did not stop.

In 2003 she had progressed to secondary progressive MS. She began taking chemotherapy drugs.

With MS, over time, the brain shrinks. This is also true with Huntington's, Parkinson's, and Alzheimer's. In looking at the latest research for these diseases, she found that they had a common theme: mitochondrial dysfunction. Mitochondria are the "power houses" of the cell. She began taking supplements that were supposed to support mitochondrial health. There were fish oil, creatine, and coenzyme Q. She continued to decline, but more slowly.

In 2007, she was so tired that she couldn't sit up anymore. She started using a zero-gravity chair.

The next thing she tried was electrical stimulation therapy. That helped.

She also discovered the Institute for Functional Medicine. She added many more vitamins and supplements. She took these for 6 months but did not feel any difference. She decided to quit taking them. Over the next few days, she felt extreme fatigue. She started taking them again. She felt much better. She tried this a few more times until she was convinced that the vitamins were making a big difference. She was feeling better.

Her physicians had told her that once an ability was lost, it never came back, so she had little hope of ever walking again. She did not expect to reverse her disease. She was just trying to stop the progression.

The next change she made was to get the nutrition from real food rather than supplements. She asked her doctors what she should be eating to match the vitamin supplements. Interestingly, they did not know. Physicians are typically not trained in nutrition. Where did she find this information? The internet. Google knew.

She began eating:

- greens
- sulfur-rich vegetables
- deeply colored vegetables and berries
- grass-fed meat
- wild fish
- organ meat
- seaweed

She got dramatic results from this!! She reports:

"That is when the magic began to happen. The following month, my energy was much better and the brain fog was gone. Two months later, I was walking between exam rooms using a cane. Six months later, I rode my bike for the first time in nearly six years. At 9 months, I completed an 18-mile bike ride with my family. My world had completely changed."

She was getting better!! No one who had MS had ever recovered a function once it was lost. She was making history!!

She says,

"I am grateful for having MS. It is one of the most profound gifts I ever received. Now I know that diet and lifestyle can be utterly transformative. We can all embrace health for ourselves, our families, our communities, our countries, our world. We can all grow younger, stronger, healthier, even sexier, by eating a deeply nutrient-dense diet, giving our cells what they need to heal and thrive. If I can make these profound changes to my heath, imagine what you could do for yours."

This is the list of things she recommends to be healthy:

1. Go gluten free.
2. Eat and live organic.
3. Eat a plate of greens each day. These can be cooked or raw. She recommends 9 cups per day.
4. Eat a plate of sulfur-rich vegetables each day. Sulfur-rich

vegetables include cabbage, onion, garlic, asparagus, broccoli, cauliflower, kale, mushrooms and Brussels sprouts.

5. Eat a rainbow each day (red, yellow, orange, and purple). Both vegetables and fruit.

6. Eat grass-fed meat and wild fish.

7. Eat seaweed once a week.

8. Eat organ meat once a week.

9. Meditate.

10. Exercise.

She says she eats 9 cups of vegetables per day. However, she is 6' tall, so maybe 6 cups of vegetables might be right for a smaller woman.

Some things she recommends that may be different from other health experts: no wheat, no dairy, no eggs, no beans. Eat seaweed and organ meat once a week.

Impressive story!!

I recommend you watch her Ted Talk. [136]

Is she cured of MS? No. She says that if she eats something she should not eat, she feels it within 24 hours, and it typically takes 2 weeks to go away. She still has MS, but she is symptom-free as long as she sticks to her program.

Is MS a genetic disease? Yes and no. Yes, in that there are a few hundred genes that contribute to the possibility of MS. Each gene incrementally adds to that possibility. However, it is not a genetic disease in that if we take care of ourselves, we may never know that we have the genes.

Bottom line, her diet is an excellent example of what to eat.

She has eliminated most things that people tend to have a bad reaction to (grains, dairy and beans).

She has eliminated what research has shown to be toxic foods (sugar, vegetable oils, and refined grains).

She includes most of the things we need to provide our bodies with, and the range of nutrition we need to be in excellent health (grass-fed meats, a range of vegetables and fruits).

Interesting facts:

How much processed or packaged food can you eat in a week and still be fine? (Hot dogs, fries, pizza, burgers, candy, cookies, cokes,

etc.)

Terry Wahls says that if she eats even one thing, she feels it within 24 hours and it takes up to 2 weeks for the effects to go away.

Suzanne Summers has written 25 books. She had cancer in 2001, and has had other health problems. She says that she has a sugar sensitivity. She has completely eliminated sugar. If she has even one date, she has a reaction.

Autism

Daniel Amen

Daniel Amen, M.D., is a psychiatrist who has scanned 120,000 brains and came up with a protocol to cure unhealthy brains. He scans brains, does his intervention, then re-scans the brain to see what changed.

Dr. Amen has seen over 1,000 patients with an Autism Spectrum Disorder (ASD). He has concluded that there are 8-10 different factors that influence abnormal brain function.

Brains can be overactive or under-active. Even if you don't know exactly what kind of autism you or your loved one might have, he recommends that we eliminate anything that can hurt the brain.

Food has a profound impact on our health. According to Dr. Amen, with regard to autism, what are the foods that most damage the brain? [137]

- **Dairy.** Dr. Amen says that, "when people with ASD removed dairy from their diet, they began talking more, their hyperactivity was reduced, and bowel problems were resolved."
- **Gluten.** Gluten is found mainly in wheat, rye, and barley. Grains are often sprayed with poison at the end of growing to make them ready to harvest, so there is the additional issue of glyphosate poison in the grain.
- **Corn.** Eighty-five percent of the corn raised in the United States is raised with pesticides.
- **Sugar.** Avoiding sugar and refined carbohydrates, and increasing lean protein can dramatically improve concentration and judgment, and decrease impulsiveness.
- **Artificial Ingredients.** While these things are not really foods, they are in so many packaged products. Avoid all additives, preservatives, dyes and artificial colors, artificial flavorings, and

artificial sweeteners.

Dr. Natasha Campbell-McBride

Dr. Campbell-McBride says that autism was I in 10,000 in the Western world 20 years ago. Now in Britain it is one child in 66. She says the numbers are similar in America, Australia and New Zealand. In Hungary it is now close to one child in 150.

In her book, *Gut and Psychology Syndrome,*[99] she describes the connection between the functioning of the gut and the functioning of the brain. She believes that autistic children are born with normal healthy brains and nervous systems. The issue is that their gut microbiome do not develop normally. As a result, their gut flora, instead of being a source of nutrition for the developing child, becomes a source of toxicity.

Because of the lack of healthy gut flora, their gut lining doesn't stay intact. Toxins leak into the body and into the brain. Their brains don't work well. In particular, they have trouble with sensory information. Because they are not getting adequate sensory information, they don't learn things about the world as other babies do.

Breastfeeding provides some protection for the babies. For breastfed babies, autism usually begins in the second year of life. For babies that are not breastfed, autism may begin earlier.

Depending on how severe the problem is with the gut flora, the child may develop autism, or maybe attention deficit hyperactivity disorder (ADHD), or attention deficit disorder (ADD) or dyslexia, or dyspraxia or obsessive-compulsive disorder, or a mixture of all of these.

Why is this happening? When did it begin? Dr. Campbell-McBride believes that it began with the use of antibiotics. Living in us are several ecosystems of bacteria, viruses, yeasts, worms and protozoa. We need these to be healthy. Antibiotics wipe out many of the beneficial bacteria.

Also living in us are thousands of species of pathogenic bacteria, fungi, viruses, and other microbes. As long as there are enough healthy species of microbes, they keep the pathogenic ones under control.

What creates this problem with the gut flora?

- Every course of antibiotics wipes out healthy microbes and gives the pathogenic microbes a chance to take over.
- Taking contraceptives also kills gut bacteria.

- Eating junk foods and processed carbohydrates feed the unhealthy bacteria.

Other illnesses may begin at this time from having unhealthy gut flora, such as diabetes type 1, celiac disease, asthma, eczema, or various autoimmune diseases.

Our gut microbiome is a major part of our immune system, so, for children who have unhealthy gut flora, their immune system is compromised.

This is why vaccinations are a problem. If these children already have compromised immune systems, their little bodies cannot handle so many disease bacteria being introduced in the form of vaccines.

Dr. Campbell-McBride has developed a protocol to reverse autism. It has three parts.

First is diet. She considers that autism is primarily a digestive disorder. She says that it takes two years for healthy gut flora to be established, and to heal the damaged gut lining. She focuses on foods that are rich in nutrition and are easy to digest.

She says, "They will never return to the terrible Western junk diet because the Western diet is absolutely terrible. What people are eating on a daily basis is appalling." [138]

The second part of the protocol is probiotics and vitamin supplements in order to introduce a healthy range of bacteria.

The third part of the protocol is detoxification for such things as mercury, lead, arsenic, and various other toxic chemicals in our environment today.

She recommends the following diet:
Eliminate these:

- Sugars
- All starches including wheat, rye, rice, oats, millet, quinoa, couscous, amaranth, buckwheat, corn and all beans.
- Milk (because of the lactose)
- Vegetable oils (coconut oil is fine)

The only sweeteners she allows are raw honey and dried fruits.

What does she recommend eating?

- All meats, fish and shellfish
- Vegetables
- Fruits
- Nuts
- Oily seeds such as sunflower, pumpkin and sesame seeds.

When people are beginning the diet, she suggests that they eliminate all fiber, all raw fruits and vegetables, and all nuts.

Meat stock, bone broth, and cooked vegetables are the core of this introductory diet. In order to introduce healthy bacteria, she also recommends fermented foods.

She says that this diet is also good for anyone who suffers from digestive issues, such as ulcerative colitis. [138]

Alzheimer's

The number one concern of individuals as we age is the loss of our cognitive abilities.

Dale Bredesen, M.D. [83]

Dr. Mary Newport

I first came across the idea that Alzheimer's can be reversed from reading about Dr. Mary Newport. Her husband, Steve, at 58, had severe Alzheimer's that had gradually been getting worse over the previous 5 years. This was in 2008. She had heard of a clinical trial that gave Alzheimer's patients MCT (medium chain triglyceride) oil in an attempt to reverse Alzheimer's. Her husband did not qualify for the trial, so she tried doing it herself. MCT oil comes from coconut oil, so she decided to give him 2 tbsp of coconut oil per day (she later gave him more). She saw results that day.

The theory is that Alzheimer's patients lose their ability to use glucose. However, our cells can use ketones as well as glucose. The coconut oil provides them with an immediate supply of ketones, so the brain, just a few hours after consuming the coconut oil, begins to function better.

He got progressively better over the next few months. Dr. Newport put the information on the internet, and many other people tried using MCT oil. Now the caregivers of many Alzheimer's patients are reporting impressive improvement with MCT oil therapy.

Research shows that over half of the people who take MCT oil show improvement.

The ketones peak about 3 hours after ingesting coconut oil, and last for up to 7 hours. Multiple doses throughout the day may be required. It's best to start with a small amount in the beginning. It can cause stomach upset of you if you start with a large dose.

There are many other diseases that respond to ketone therapy including ALS, Lou Gehrig's, Parkinson's, autism, seizures, and epilepsy. [139]

Dr. Bredesen

One of the most interesting books on Alzheimer's is *The End of Alzheimer's,* written by Dr. Bredesen, published in 2017. Dr. Bredesen has developed a protocol that he has used to cure Alzheimer's. [83]

The following are the highlights of his book. *My additions are in italics.*

What you need to know about Alzheimer's:

- When you first experience symptoms, you have probably had it for at least 20 years.
- There are about 36 different contributing factors to Alzheimer's.
- All contributing factors need to be addressed to reverse or cure the disease.
- There is no pill that can do this job.
- The medical profession still largely believes that Alzheimer's is incurable and unstoppable (there is nothing you can do).

The truth is that Alzheimer's can be reversed and/or cured, especially in the early stages for most people.

For a thorough scientific explanation, I recommend reading his book. For a great summary of his book, I recommend watching his lectures on YouTube.

What are some of the first symptoms of Alzheimer's?

- Difficulty recognizing and remembering faces
- Decreasing mental clarity
- Decreasing interest in reading

- Inability to follow or engage in complex conversations
- Inability to follow movies with complicated plots
- Difficulty completing tasks
- Decreasing ability to recall what is read or heard
- Decreasing vocabulary or difficulty coming up with the right word
- Mixing up words
- Decreasing processing speed
- Increasing anxiety about driving (forgetting where you are going)
- Difficulty remembering appointments

As it progresses, people may experience:

- Feeling overwhelmed about what there is to do.
- Sleep disruption. Difficulty going to sleep. Easily waking up. Difficulty going back to sleep, waking up many times during the night.
- Confusion with time and place
- Decreased judgment, especially about financial matters.
- Changes in mood (may be confused, leading to anxiety, irritability, anger or fear)
- Hesitant to try new things
- Withdrawal from social activities

This is a summary of the protocol he has developed:

Food: When and what to eat.

- Ketogenic diet. He recommends 12 hours between dinner and breakfast. Some people may need to fast up to 16 hours to produce results. Wait at least 3 hours between your last meal and going to bed. To review what ketosis is: we burn either glucose or ketones. We burn glucose after we eat. We burn ketones when we have finished burning glucose (usually about 8 hours after eating), or when we eat fat and severely limit carbohydrate intake. Having some period of mild ketosis is important for optimal health.
- Primarily eat foods with a glycemic index lower than 35.
- Avoid fruit juices. Eat whole fruit instead.
- Avoid simple carbohydrates.
- Avoid saturated fats. (This is not what many other researchers

suggest)

- Avoid gluten and dairy. He says that many people have allergies to these things. These could be contributing to leaky gut and inflammation.
- Cleanse your body of toxins by eating certain plants. These are: cilantro, avocadoes, artichokes, beets, dandelions, garlic, ginger, grapefruit, lemons, olive oil, seaweed and cruciferous vegetables (cauliflower, broccoli, cabbage, kale, radishes, Brussels sprouts, turnips, watercress, kohlrabi, rutabaga, arugula, horseradish, maca, and bok choy).
- Eat healthy fats such as avocadoes, nuts, seeds, olive oil, and MCT oil.
- Avoid processed foods. What is a processed food? Anything with a label. Eat fresh, local, sustainable, organic vegetables.
- Fish are optional. Fish are an excellent source of omega 3's and protein. However, some fish have high mercury content and other contaminants. He suggests SMASH fish (salmon, mackerel, anchovies, sardines, and herring). These fish have short lives (limiting mercury exposure). Avoid fish with long lives, such as sharks, swordfish, and tuna.
- Eat meat as a condiment, not the main course. Eat chicken that is pasture-fed chicken, and grass-fed beef. Eat 2-3 oz a few nights per week, at most. Eggs should be from pasture-fed chickens.
- Include probiotics and prebiotics. Probiotics are fermented foods such as kimchi, sauerkraut, sour pickles, miso soup, and kombucha. He suggests avoiding yogurt because it is a dairy product and contains sugar (lactose), even though it is a probiotic.
- He includes digestive enzymes, supplements, and herbs in capsule form. They are listed in his book.
- Do not cook on high heat. High heat may damage the nutritional value of your food.

Exercise. Why do it?

- Reduces insulin resistance
- Increases ketosis
- Increases the size of the hippocampus, a key region for memory
- Increases vascular function
- Reduces stress
- Improves sleep

- Increases the survival of new neurons
- Improves mood

Dr. Bredesen suggests combining aerobic exercise (walking, running, dancing, or spinning) with weight training, at lease 4-5 hours per week, 45-60 minutes each day.

Sleep. He suggests a minimum of 8 hours per night without sleeping pills.

Reduce stress

Brain training. He suggests various computer-based programs for keeping your brain sharp.

Reduce inflammation

Heal the gut. Leaky gut is very common. If you have food sensitivities, bloating, constipation, or loose stools, you probably have leaky gut. This means that the integrity of your gut lining has been compromised. The bacteria in your intestines are crucial for nutrient absorption, production of hormones and neurotransmitters

This is a list of potential causes of leaky gut:

- Sugar
- Gluten
- Dairy
- Processed foods
- Herbicides *(such as glyphosate)*
- Pesticides
- GMO foods *(Genetically Modified Organisms)*
- Alcohol
- Antibiotics
- Anti-inflammatories such as aspirin or ibuprofen or steroids
- Stress

Toxins

- General anesthesia (toxic chemicals and possible oxygen deprivation)

- Dental amalgams (mercury poisoning)
- Eating fish high in mercury
- Certain medications, especially those that influence brain function, such as Valium, antidepressants, blood pressure pills, statins, proton pump inhibitors, or antihistamines
- Using street drugs
- Drinking alcohol
- Smoking cigarettes
- Bad oral hygiene, causing chronic inflammation in body
- Surgical implants
- Consuming hot-pressed oils (heat may degrade oils and therefore damage your brain)
- Eating trans fats or refined carbohydrates (vascular damage and insulin resistance)
- Chronic sinus problems (possible mold exposure)
- Toxic mold in your home, car, or workplace
- Eating processed foods or nonorganic foods (insulin resistance or toxic exposure)
- Tick bites (lime disease and other pathogens leading to chronic inflammation)
- Makeup, hair spray, or antiperspirants (toxic exposure)
- Don't sweat much (sweat helps remove toxins)
- Constipation (bowel movements eliminate toxins)
- Not enough purified water (urine removes toxins)
- Dr. Bredesen believes that any of these might also be contributing factors to Alzheimer's:
- Head trauma, such as football and auto accidents
- Having liver, kidney, lung or heart disease
- Snoring (possibly having sleep apnea)
- Gastrointestinal problems such as bloating or recurring diarrhea (possible leaky gut)
- Proton pump inhibitors for reflux (reducing stomach acid needed for digestion and therefore reducing the uptake of zinc, vitamin B12, and other nutrients)

By leveraging 36 healthy lifestyle parameters, Dr. Bredesen was able to reverse Alzheimer's in 9 of 10 patients!! (Mercola, 2017) **Pretty amazing for a disease that the medical community commonly considers to be irreversible and incurable.**

Other thoughts about Alzheimer's

Dr. Perlmutter, author of *Grain Brain*, [140] offers a simpler explanation of the cause of Alzheimer's disease:

"[Alzheimer's] is a preventable disease. It surprises me at my core that no one's talking about the fact that so many of these devastating neurological problems are, in fact, modifiable based upon lifestyle choices . . . What we've crystallized it down to now, in essence, is that diets that are high in sugar and carbohydrates, and similarly diets that are low in fat, are devastating to the brain. When you have a diet that has carbohydrates in it, you are paving the way for Alzheimer's disease. I want to be super clear about that. Dietary carbohydrates lead to Alzheimer's disease. It's a pretty profound statement, but it's empowering nonetheless when we realize that we control our diet. We control our choices, whether to favor fat or carbohydrates." [141]

Dr. Joseph Mercola, author of *KetoFast*, [18] says,

"A high-fat, moderate-protein, low net-carb ketogenic diet is crucial for preventing degeneration that can lead to Alzheimer's. High-carb diets have been shown to increase your risk of dementia by 89% while high-fat diets lower it by 44%."

Acne

Acne may not seem like such an important disease to include here, but it has an unusual characteristic: it can be easily seen. We can't see heart disease, or diabetes, or cancer, but we can see acne. We can see if it is getting better or worse. In addition, acne responds very quickly to changes in our diet, and we can readily see these changes.

In addition, if your skin is having a problem, chances are that you are having problems inside your body, too. Your skin can give you such clear feedback about the general health of your body.

Acne is controlled by diet

Acne seems to be nearly universal among American teenagers. However, it is not universal among other humans. There are many groups around the world who do not experience acne at all. Why is that? Is it a genetic difference? Evidence suggests that it is diet, not genes.

Acne-free populations include:

- The Kitavans of New Guinea who exist on a hunter-gatherer diet of vegetables, fruits, tubers, coconuts, and fish.
- The Paraguayan Ache hunter-gatherers, who eat a similar diet but add land animals and cultivated manioc, peanuts, rice, and maize.
- Japanese Okinawans, until the 1980's, consumed a diet of vegetables, sweet potatoes, soy, pork, and fish. [142]
- The traditional Inuit diet, consisted of seal, fish, caribou, seaweed, berries and roots.
- African Bantus and Zulus ate a variety of wild plants such as guava, mangoes, and tomatoes, and also fish and wild game. [143]

Notice that the cultures without acne do not consume wheat, sugar, or dairy products. [85]

As Western foods are introduced, acne begins, along with all of the other diseases we have talked about. [144] [145] [146] This makes it quite clear that it is not genetic.

Interestingly, it was commonly accepted in the early twentieth century that starchy foods (bread and pancakes) caused or at least contributed to acne. [85]

Currently, modern dermatologists focus on reducing the symptoms of acne with medication, just as other specialties focus on symptom removal through drugs. Even with something as visible as the skin, we do not deal with the cause of the problem.

Exactly how does food cause acne?

"Insulin stimulates the release of a hormone called insulin-like growth factor-1, or IGF-1, within the skin. IGF-1, in turn stimulates tissue growth in the hair follicles and in the dermis, the layer of skin just beneath the surface. Insulin and IGF-1 also stimulate the production of sebum, the oily protective film produced by the sebaceous glands. Overproduction of sebum along with skin tissue growth, leads to the characteristic upward-growing reddened pimple." [85]

In addition to starches causing acne, milk also seems to add to the problem. It's not the fat. It is a protein in milk. Teenagers who consume milk have a 20 percent increase in acne. [147]

I think the lactose (sugar) may contribute to the problem.

If starches cause acne, then all we have to do is change the diet and acne disappears, or at least is reduced. Does this happen? Yes!

A group of college students, in a randomized controlled trial, were told to eat a low-glycemic diet or a high glycemic diet for 12 weeks. Participants who cut their carbohydrate intake the most reduced the acne lesions by 50 percent. [148]

We can control acne with diet. If we eliminate high-glycemic foods (sugar, wheat, crackers, tortillas, chips, bagels, pancakes, and even whole wheat bread), acne should disappear.

For a more thorough review of this information, read *Wheat Belly* by William Davis. [85]

Personal Note

When I was a teenager, my mother banned wheat and sugar and potatoes from our household. I had very clear skin. Once a week, I went to a meeting that served cookies after the gathering. If I ate a cookie, my face would break out within a few days. Was it the sugar, flour, or maybe the processed oils? I didn't know, but I did know that the cookies caused the breakouts. Because of this, I rarely ate the cookies, even though I liked sweets, just like other teenagers do. But I liked to have clear skin more. I can see now that my clear skin was not genetic. It was from the choices I made.

Another Personal Story

I went to a coed summer camp when I was 18 years old. One of the adult male counselors (who had severe acne scars) was watching us as we washed our faces and brushed our teeth. Afterward, he came up to me and said, "You wash your faced with Dial soap?! I don't understand how you can have such beautiful skin if that is all you do." I did wash my face with Dial soap as a teenager. I also used some inexpensive face cream. Again, I don't think it is the expensive face treatments that make most of the difference. It is primarily food, sleep, exercise, attitude, etc. that matter. That said, I do use a face cream for aging skin. Just in case.

Digestive disorders:

What are digestive disorders?

- Bloating
- Abdominal pain
- Diarrhea
- Constipation
- Underweight or overweight
- Acid reflux
- Heartburn
- Nutritional deficiencies
- Leaky gut
- IBS (irritable bowel syndrome)
- Celiac disease (sensitivity to gluten)
- Ulcerative colitis
- GERD (gastroesophageal reflux disease)
- Allergies and food sensitivities
- Gastrointestinal infections

There are two excellent books on this subject. If you have any of these issues, I recommend that you read:

- *Gut and Physiology Syndrome: Natural Treatment for Allergies, Autoimmune Illness, Arthritis, Gut Problems, Fatigue, Hormonal Problems, Neurological Disease and More* by Natasha Campbell-McBride, M.D. [138] and
- *Digestive Health with Real food a practical guide to an anti-inflammatory, low-irritant, nutrient-dense diet for IBS and other digestive issues* by Aglaee Jacob, M.S., R.D. [149]

The first is more scientific, and the second is very thorough.

They both suggest being on an elimination diet of primarily bone broth, meat and animal fat until the symptoms go away, then slowly add one vegetable at a time and see how your body reacts.

(Personal Note)

I think that many people have digestive systems that are ongoingly irritated, but they don't pay much attention to it. They think it is "normal". I suggest that you try eating healthy food until you feel really good. I predict that you will then start to notice the difference if you go off your healthy diet.

Why Isn't My Doctor Telling Me This?

"Doctors don't get taught much about nutrition, but the real problem is that what little we do get taught is mostly wrong. . . Doctors are parroting guidelines about what they get taught in medical school, to the detriment, I believe, of the health of our population."
--Dr. Paul Mason, [87]

"What medical students aren't being taught is: if you fix the root cause, which is diet and lifestyle, you could roll back these progressive diseases."
--Dr. Terry Wahls [150]

"We are getting fatter and sicker. That is the problem. How did we get here? . . . In medicine, we have believed that nutrition science is the same as medical science, but it is not. It is a shambles and we are now waking up to that. . . We can't wait. . . We can't wait for governments to change policy because they are influenced by lobbyists. We can't wait for industry to change, or corporations to change because they are driven by profit. We can't wait for the health professionals to change because they are all following guidelines . . . there is a fear of coming out and talking about this. We need to do something now."
--Gary Fettke [151]

Who becomes a doctor? Typically, they are among the smartest kids in every high school. They could probably do anything with their lives and be successful. They become doctors because they are smart, hard-working, dedicated people who want to do something important with their lives. We are lucky they have chosen to be our doctors.

However, doctors are not trained in nutrition, or if they are, it is very minimal, or even worse, they are given information that is just plain wrong.

They are terrific with acute illnesses. If you break a leg, they are great at fixing it.

However, if you have a chronic illness, **they are trained to diagnose, then medicate. Rarely does this system "cure" the illness. It just masks the symptoms.**

Dr. Sten Ekberg on YouTube does a great job of describing our current medical system. He says our medical system primarily addresses symptoms, not the cause of the illness.

The following is my version of his analogy.

Pretend you are driving a car. The overheating light comes on. What you should do is pull over and find out why the light came on. Perhaps the radiator is out of water. Is a water hose leaking? If so, repair the hose, fill the radiator with water, and continue driving, and maybe keep a careful eye on the overheating light.

Instead, what our medical system does is get rid of the symptom. In our analogy, that means that we have a handy roll of duct tape with us. When a light comes on, we get our tape out and cover up the light.

If another light comes on, perhaps the oil light, we pull out our handy duct tape and cover up that light. If we do this with our medical symptoms, we really should not wonder why we continue to get sicker and sicker. We need to address the cause of the illness and fix that if we expect to get better.

For example, let's look at **cancer.**

You go to the doctor with a lump. They test the lump. If it is cancer, the options are:

- Surgery
- Chemotherapy
- Radiation

They probably don't talk about cancer being a lifestyle disease, and one possibility is to treat it with changes in how you live your life. Perhaps you could eat healthier food, or improve your sleep, or reduce stress. They probably don't say that most cancers need glucose to live, but the rest of your cells can live on glucose or ketones, so one way to reverse cancer is to get your body to burn ketones more often. This starves the cancer. This isn't part of standard training.

If you are eating sugar, wheat flour, processed oils, processed and packaged foods, don't exercise, are overweight, are depressed, under stress, don't sleep well, smoke, drink too much alcohol, or any combination of these things, eventually it is likely that you will get sick.

What illness? That is where your genes come into play. Your genetic weak spot will show up here. However, if you take care of yourself, you will probably never know what your weak gene is. You will simply be healthy.

Let's look at **heart disease.**

You get dizzy when you stand up. You go to the doctor. What does he do? Lots of tests followed by:

- Medication?
- Surgery?

The doctor probably does say that you should "eat less and exercise more". This does not work (see chapter on your ideal weight) Or maybe your doctor will refer you to a nutritionist. However, the nutritionist will probably direct you to the government guidelines which are the very recommendations that created the problem to begin with.

It is not all the doctor's fault. The society has the attitude that we get to live however we want: eating junk food every day, not exercising, and not taking care of our bodies. If we get sick, the doctor will have a pill to take care of it.

A word about medications

Forty-four percent of Americans take one prescription drug, and 17% take three or more. In the population over 65, five out of six people take at least one prescription medication, and half of those over 65 take 3 or more medications.

Again, half of people over 65 take three or more prescription medications!

What effect are these medications having on us?

Let's look at aspirin. When I was a child, that was the "go-to" medication. If we had headaches or aches and pains, we took an aspirin.

Most of our current "fancy" drugs did not exist back then.

What does aspirin do? It reduces pain. But what else does it do? It keeps blood from coagulating. That's why some people are told to take baby aspirin daily to prevent heart attacks (which can be a problem if you need emergency surgery, and your blood won't coagulate). What else? It irritates the stomach and can cause bleeding in the stomach lining.

All of that from the simple little aspirin.

What are all of these "fancy" medications doing to us? We don't really know. Each medication has its own side effects, and combined, there are more side effects from drug interactions.

The population of Americans is a huge science experiment. There are the GMO foods we are eating, all of the packaged and processed "foods" that have so many odd ingredients, poisons in our food, air and water, and now add: the unknown effects of the medications we are taking.

Wow! We, as a country, are getting sicker and sicker, but there are so many possibilities about what is causing it.

I suggest that you take a look at the medications you are taking and consider eliminating them. One by one. Slowly. Under a doctor's supervision. But eliminate them.

Make yourself healthy the old-fashioned way: with changes in your lifestyle.

Note: I am not a physician. I am not giving medical advice. I am giving a suggestion for you to consider.

Personal Note

When I was in my 20's, I had a minor rash on my face. I went to the doctor, and was given a prescription for cortisone cream. It did get rid of the rash. The doctor kept giving me more prescriptions. If I missed applying it in the morning, I had a really terrible rash just that afternoon, much worse than the original rash.

Finally, I decided that I needed to solve this problem in a better way. I stopped using the cortisone cream. I had a really terrible rash for about a week. It was much, much worse than my original rash. After the week of "withdrawal" from the cortisone cream, I was back to my mild rash.

I thought about what could be causing a rash on my face. My face cream? I changed to a new face cream. That wasn't it. My face soap? I changed that. That wasn't it. Finally, I tried changing my laundry detergent. That was it! Just using the towel to dry my face was enough to cause the rash. I was allergic to something in that particular laundry detergent (It was a popular national brand).

The doctor never asked me any questions to find out what might be causing the rash. He just gave me the prescription.

My point is that you cannot count on doctors to figure out what to do. They are often in such a hurry that they don't take the time to ask you very many questions. Also, they are trained to reduce or eliminate symptoms, not to look for the cause of the problem.

You need to be in charge of your own health. No one else will care as much as you do.

American Medical Association Guidelines

If I were to sum up the views of the AMA toward diet, it would be: Go ahead and eat sugar and foods that increase blood sugar, just be sure to adjust your medication to compensate.
-- William Davis, M.D. [85]

The AMA advises diabetics to cut fat, reduce saturated fat, and include 45 to 60 grams of carbohydrates -- preferably "healthy whole grains" -- in each meal. Or 135 to 180 grams of carbohydrates per day, not including snacks. It is, in essence, a fat-phobic, carbohydrate-centered diet, with 55 to 65 percent of calories from carbohydrates.
-- William Davis, M.D. [85]

If doctors do get information about what food to eat, it may be incorrect information.

What are some of the AMA-recommended foods?

- Whole grain breads, such as whole wheat or rye
- Whole grain, high-fiber cereal

- Cooked cereal such as oatmeal, grits, hominy, or cream of wheat
- Rice, pasta, tortillas
- Potatoes, green peas, corn, lima beans
- Low-fat crackers and snack chips, pretzels, and fat-free popcorn [85]

Eating food that is high in carbohydrates is exactly how we got into this health mess. If the AMA is recommending these very unhealthy foods, can you really blame the doctors for accepting these guidelines and passing that information on to you?

American Heart Association recommendations

Let's take a look at what the American Heart Association suggests.

The American Heart Association wrote a book called Complete guide to Women's Heart Health, published in 2009. [152]

These are some of statements from the book.

See if you can figure out what the problem is with each of these statements:

AHA statement: "Your liver produces the cholesterol in your blood. If your liver produces a high level of LDL cholesterol (the "bad" cholesterol), that excess contributes to a process called atherosclerosis."

Answer: Your liver does produce most of the cholesterol for your body.

Cholesterol only acts like a "band aid" to the inflamed artery walls. The real culprit is not "excess cholesterol" but the spiking and crashing of your blood sugar, creating problems with your artery walls (see full explanation above on heart disease) Also, only the small dense LDL particles are harmful, not the large, fluffy LDL particles. In addition, people with high cholesterol live the longest, which puts into question the whole idea of "excess cholesterol".

AHA statement: "Aim for about 25 grams of fiber a day, with at least half that amount coming from whole grains."

Answer: Fiber is good for us, and 25 grams is a good minimum. Grains are in the "questionable" group of foods. Many people have an adverse reaction to grains. In addition, most grains spike blood sugar, which is a primary driver of our diseases. The best way to increase fiber is to eat non-starchy vegetables

AHA statement: "To lose weight, eat only 75 percent of the amount of food you normally eat, or substitute lower-calorie foods for the high-calorie foods you eat regularly. For example, if you are used to buying a cinnamon roll on your way to work, try toasting a cinnamon-raisin English muffin at home instead and save yourself about 300 calories."

Answer: Wow! This is bad advice on so many levels. First of all, if you just eat less, you will probably be hungry. Will power can only last for so long. The real solution is to eat more fats and perhaps more protein. They leave you feeling full longer. In addition, the solution is to limit or eliminate sugar and processed foods like flour. To suggest eating a smaller version of unhealthy food is not helpful. It will still spike blood sugar, then blood sugar will crash. Hunger and fatigue will follow. Your metabolism will slow down as time goes on to compensate for the reduced caloric intake. In the end, you will not lose weight.

AHA statement: They recommend eating "fat-free and low-fat dairy products".

Answer: We are meant to eat food just as it comes to us. I recommend full-fat dairy products. Fat keeps us full longer, and we need fat for our brains and to fuel our bodies. The casein, a protein in milk might be a problem. Some research has found it to be carcinogenic. Another part of milk is lactose (sugar). This could cause a spike in insulin. In addition, many people have problems digesting lactose, and may need to eliminate dairy altogether. The healthiest part of the milk is the fat. Also, there is no mention of "grass-fed" dairy products being healthier.

AHA statement: "Fortified ready-to-eat cereals are recommended to get enough calcium."

Answer: Do not eat ready-to-eat cereals! They usually contain sugar, flour and artificial ingredients. They are calories, and not much else of value. We are meant to get our nutrients from real food. Instead, eat real foods that are high in calcium, such as nuts, seeds, and broccoli.

AHA statement: "Make breakfast part of your routine. Breakfast revs up your energy level and keeps your metabolism going."

Answer: In order to help your body clean out unhealthy cells, let your body have a break from digestion for 12-20 hours per day (12 at a minimum and 16 is probably adequate). The easiest way to do this is to stop eating early in the evening, and skip breakfast. We do not need breakfast. Our bodies will burn ketones rather than glucose. Our brains and bodies prefer ketones. The need for breakfast was made up by the breakfast cereal companies.

AHA statement: For people in their 70's it is recommended that we add horseshoes as an exercise.

Answer: Please! People can be physically active into their 90's, and certainly they can be active in their 70's. I suppose horseshoes is better than sitting on the couch. However, for people who have trouble moving, they might try swimming or water aerobics. They are easy on the joints, and almost everyone can do them. Walking is also a good place to begin.

AHA statement: "Science has shown that the simple formula of calories in = calories out is the best approach to maintaining your weight."

Answer: Calories do matter to some extent. If you eat unlimited amounts of high-calorie foods, you will probably gain weight. However, the "calories in = calories out" idea became popular because the sugar industries wanted you to eat sugar instead of fat. Sugar is lower in calories per tablespoon than fat. However, fat is very filling and leaves you full for many hours. Your body needs fat. It does not need sugar. Eating sugar spikes blood sugar, and very soon after eating, your blood sugar crashes, and you are hungry again. This leads to weight gain. In addition, sugar is the primary food responsible for many of our diseases. Primitive cultures were not fat, and they did not count calories. They just ate real food. See chapter on the science of weight loss for a more complete explanation.

AHA statement: "The first approach to treatment for high triglycerides is lifestyle change: lose weight if needed, reduce your intake of saturated and trans fats and dietary cholesterol, avoid alcohol, eat a balanced diet, and make regular physical activity part of your routine."

Answer: What is good and what is bad? Can you tell?

Good part:

- Lifestyle changes to lower triglycerides
- Lose weight if needed
- Avoid alcohol (which is processed like sugar)
- Eat a balanced diet (actually very vague)
- Physical activity

Bad part:

- Reduce your intake of saturated and trans fats and dietary cholesterol.

It should say: reducing or eliminating sugar, flour, and starchy carbs will reduce triglycerides. No trans fats should ever be eaten. Eating foods high in cholesterol is good for us.

AHA statement: Three treatment options are offered for coronary heart disease:

- "Reducing pain and other symptoms with medication
- Opening blocked arteries with angioplasty and stents, atherectomy, and laser ablation
- Providing a new route around blocked arteries with coronary artery bypass surgery"

Answer: The first place to begin is a change in lifestyle, not medication and surgery. Medication and surgery should only be done as a last resort. In addition, research indicates that if you change your diet and lifestyle adequately, you probably won't need medication or surgery. People can be brought back from death's door with lifestyle changes, as Esselstyn showed in 2007. [30] A change in diet and lifestyle is not even on the AHA list.

AHA statement: On a 2,000-calorie diet, trans fats should be limited to 2 grams per day.

Answer: No trans fats should ever be eaten. Even in 2002 we knew that trans fats were deadly. In 2002 the National Academy of Sciences panel reported that "the only safe intake of trans-fat is zero." [117] I think that medical advice often treats us as if we will not do what is best for us, so they recommend what they think we will be willing to do. I think it is much better to tell the truth about what is healthy and let people decide how much they are willing to do.

AHA statement: "Make it a goal to eat fatty fish, such as salmon, tuna, and trout, at least twice a week."

Answer: Yes, fatty fish are good for us, and should be eaten every week to get adequate amounts of omega 3's. However, we need to limit our mercury intake. Wild caught Alaskan Sockeye salmon is an excellent choice. It lives a short life and primarily eats algae. Farmed salmon is not a good choice. They are typically fed corn and soy (high in omega 6's, and may be contaminated with herbicides and pesticides) and may be given antibiotics and growth hormones. Tuna live a long life, therefore they eat smaller fish for many years, accumulating more and more mercury, so eating tuna is not a good choice. I see mixed reports on trout. It depends on where they are caught. They may have many of the same problems as farmed salmon.

What do you think? Should you blindly believe the guidelines of the American Heart Association?

If your doctor follows the recommendations of the American Heart Association, he or she may not be giving you good advice. Remember that you are in charge of your health.

Do doctors know about this research? About sugar? About statins? About curing diseases with food?

Whenever you get any recommendation from any source, **ask yourself, why would this person be telling me this?**

We would like to think that doctors only have our best interests in mind, but there are other things driving the recommendations of doctors. What are they?

If a doctor does not recommend what is "standard practice", he or she can be sued for malpractice, and could lose his or her license. For example, if you have a high LDL score, your doctor will probably recommend that you take a statin. If your doctor does not make this recommendation, this may be grounds for malpractice.

In addition, **doctors go to continuing education seminars** in order to renew their licenses. In these continuing education seminars, you would hope that they are getting the latest real research in medicine. However, many of the classes are sponsored by drug companies who have their representatives giving speeches that the drug companies have prepared. This is why many doctors believe that statins reduce heart disease by 30%, rather than the real reduction, which is 1% (see discussion on heart disease).

Dr. Joseph Mercola describes how this misinformation happens in the medical community:

"I was one of their paid shills in the mid-1990's and so have firsthand experience on how it works. The company would pay my travel expenses and give me checks for as much as $5,000 for speaking. That may not seem like much to some people now, but thirty years ago for someone just graduating school with loads of debt, it was a major sum. It is a magnificent system, too, as you may feel that you are doing good and being paid to share your hard-earned knowledge, when the reality is that you are merely feeding the researchers' studies bought and paid for by the drug companies so they can sell more drugs.

"And then there's the insidious drug industry-sponsored 'education' that takes place in medical schools across the United States. For example, out of Harvard's 8,900 professors and lecturers, 1600 admit that they or a family member have ties to drug companies that could

bias their teaching or research. In one year alone, the pharmaceutical industry contributed more than $11.5 million to Harvard for 'research and continuing education classes.'

"This goes on in virtually every medical institution in the United States and is a massively effective way to indoctrinate budding physicians. By influencing the recognized thought leaders of medicine, drug companies can outrageously influence the entire profession – this, combined with the previously discussed marketing efforts, and their political lobbying to change the laws to their advantage. As a patient, you don't have to fall victim to these tactics. You can learn to see right through the propaganda and stop being deceived by drug company lies and deceptions.

"Chances are your doctor, even if he or she has good intentions and a desire to heal, not harm, has fallen prey to pharmaceutical marketing tactics. Most doctors simply do not have the time to research each drug, and they rely heavily on information from their pharmaceutical reps and from other 'experts,' that is, doctors who are receiving significant fees to talk about drug treatments.

"One of my main goals in sharing this information is to keep you out of the doctor's office for anything other than preventive screenings and out of the hospital for anything but acute traumas."

Dr. Mercola concludes by saying,

"You absolutely can take control of your health. It doesn't have to be in anyone's hands but your own." [153]

Dr. Steven Sinatra, a cardiologist, tells a similar story in his book *The Great Cholesterol Myth.* [33] He says:

"Most doctors today will recommend that you take a statin drug – they might even nag you to do so – if your cholesterol numbers are high. They will do so whether or not you have evidence of arterial disease and are a man or woman, and despite your age. In their minds, you prevent heart disease by lowering cholesterol.

"Once upon a time I used to believe that, too. It made sense, based on the research and information that was promoted to doctors. I believed it to the extent that I even lectured on behalf of drug makers. I was a paid consultant to some of the biggest manufacturers of statin drugs, lecturing for hefty honorariums. I became a cholesterol choirboy,

singing the refrain of high cholesterol as the big, bad villain of heart disease. Beat it down with a drug, and you cut our risks. My thinking changed years ago when I began seeing conflicting evidence among my own patients. I saw, for instance, many patients with low total cholesterol as low as 150 mg/dl! – develop heart disease."

He described doing angiograms on patients with cholesterol readings of greater than 280 mg/dl. He found that many of these patients had arteries that were perfectly healthy. In addition, he found many other doctors who were seeing the same thing. However, "these dissenting voices were drowned out by the cholesterol chorus." Dr. Sinatra says that the cholesterol paradigm appears to continue to "have the backing of the pharmaceutical and low-fat industries along with leading regulatory agencies and medical organizations." [33]

He no longer believes the "cholesterol paradigm". He "found that life can't go on without cholesterol." It is needed for so many vital processes. Almost every cell in your body needs cholesterol. We need it to make vitamin D, to make sex hormones and bile salts. It is essential for making the myelin sheath covering our nerve cells. About one quarter of our cholesterol is used in the brain. Cholesterol is needed for neural communication, and consequently, low levels of cholesterol have been linked to poorer cognitive performance. It helps fight bacteria and infections.

Dr. Sinatra also discovered that statin drugs deplete the body of CoQ10, a nutrient that is vital to the strong pumping of the heart. [33]

There are so many vital processes that need cholesterol! Why are we making it difficult for our bodies to make cholesterol by taking a statin?

Here are two doctors who believed so much in the "truth" the pharmaceutical industries put out, that they were paid lecturers, only to discover later that they were really just "paid shills" for the drug companies.

(Personal Note)

I have a high cholesterol score, so every doctor I visit suggests that I take a statin. I have high HDL (good), low triglycerides (good), low VLDL (good), but high total cholesterol because I have a high score in the large fluffy LDL (the harmless kind).

I talk about this to every doctor who recommends that I take a statin. They don't know what I am talking about. They really just don't know. Even the cardiologists I've talked to don't know these things. I believe that they are not trying to do harm. They simply follow the recommendations from the American Heart Association. **They are recommending what they are told to recommend, and what they understand to be true.**

In addition, **there is no money in people curing themselves of diseases with food. However, billions are being made by the pharmaceutical companies by selling pills to lessen the symptoms of diseases, even if these pills may be ultimately killing people.**

In addition, **billions are being made by the food manufacturers, selling us food that is killing us. They don't want the food recommendations changed.**

Follow the money.

My friend's story

I had a neighbor who had and some severe medical problems. I offered to go to with him to his medical appointments to help him understand his health conditions.

We started with his GP. We learned that the blood flow coming out of his heart was 29% (normal is 55-65%). His blood pressure is 80 over 55 (normal is about 115 over 70). This means that his heart was hardly pumping any blood, with low pressure and low volume. According to his GP, this is not enough blood flow to keep his internal organs alive. In other words, he was dying. His doctor also said that people do not recover from this. Once it is this bad, that's it. No hope.

The next day we went to see his cardiologist. He was telling my friend that he was just fine. Everything was OK. I thought this was odd, considering that his GP had just told him that he was dying, so I asked him some questions:

Me: Why are you saying that he is "fine"? The blood flow out of his heart is only 29%, and his blood pressure is 80 over 55. I don't understand.

Cardiologist: He is being managed with medication.

Me: Well, I think he needs to change the way he is eating. He needs to lose weight (he weighed 330 pounds). I don't understand why you are telling him that he is fine. If you tell him he is fine, he will have no motivation to improve his health. Please tell him the truth about the condition of his health.

Cardiologist: People never recover from these things. There is no point in upsetting him. If I say something upsetting, that creates stress and stress contributes to his heart problems. Yes, he should lose weight, but he has no motivation to do that. No one can make him.

Me: He needs to know how bad his health is, then he can make decisions about what he wants to do.

Cardiologist: No one recovers from a heart condition this bad.

Me: People can recover from severe heart problems.

Cardiologist: No they can't.

Me: We will just have to disagree on that.

Cardiologist: I have seen over 8,000 patients. No one has ever gotten better.

I left thinking that of course no one gets better. He does not tell them how bad it is. He does not believe that anyone will lose weight or change the way they are eating. He gives them no information about what they can do to be healthier, and **he does not believe that anyone can get better.**

I said to my friend after we left, "Let's prove him wrong".

He said, "OK. Let's prove him wrong."

My friend's typical eating consisted of doughnuts in the morning with coffee with several teaspoons of sugar. Then a Coke. Lunch was Wendy's or something similar.

My friend agreed to let me take all of the unhealthy things out of his apartment, such as boxes of macaroni and cheese, loaves of white bread, and boxes of sugared cereals.

We went shopping together and bought organic fruits and vegetables, and healthy meats.

Two weeks later, we went back to his GP for a follow-up visit.

My friend had lost 10 pounds, and his blood pressure was back to normal (108 over 60). Wow! This happened in just 2 weeks of healthy eating.

Four weeks later the cardiologist scheduled him for another test to check his blood flow. It was now up to 39%. In just four weeks, his blood flow had significantly improved.

His GP said that this was very unusual. He rarely sees anyone improve on their blood flow. It usually only gets worse.

A few months later, we visited the cardiologist again. At this point, my friend had lost 30 pounds. When the cardiologist saw that his blood flow had improved, and that his blood pressure was normal, and that he had lost 30 pounds, he oddly didn't say anything. He didn't ask how it improved. I think he didn't want to know. His GP didn't ask, either.

I think that many physicians simply do not believe that people can get better with diet and lifestyle changes. They do their best to manage people with medications. However, this is just managing the symptoms, rather than getting rid of the problem. Of course people don't get better with this system.

Take Away

- **Many of our chronic diseases can be prevented or reversed through food and lifestyle changes. These diseases include heart disease, cancer, diabetes, multiple sclerosis, Alzheimer's, autism, digestive disorders, acne, and many others.**
- **Americans are participating in a huge science experiment. We eat poisons and chemicals in our foods. We are eating foods that weren't even considered foods until about 100 years ago. We are breathing chemicals in contaminated air. We are drinking water with chemicals, such as fluoride and clorine. And we are also adding various medications to all of this, and then there are the interactions between medications. No wonder we are so sick!**
- **The government guidelines and all of the guidelines based on it (the AMA guidelines, the Heart Association guidelines, the American Diabetes guidelines, and the American Cancer Society guidelines) are making our health worse, not better.**

Chapter 8

Some Important Nutrients

Vitamin K2

Vitamin K2 is a very important element in our food, and comes almost exclusively from eating animals and animal products. Considering how important it is to our health, it is rather surprising how unknown it is.

We used to get plenty of vitamin K2 without even being aware of it. However, since we started feeding our animals GMO corn and soy, instead of what they would naturally be eating (grass), we get very little vitamin K2, and are suffering the consequences.

What does vitamin K2 do?

- Takes calcium where it needs to go (to bones and teeth and not to arteries)
- Heals scars
- Reduces wrinkles
- Prevents varicose veins
- Increases exercise performance
- Helps prevent kidney stones

- Helps prevent cancer by regulating cell growth
- Vital for brain function and preventing degenerative disease
- Helps prevent mitochondrial dysfunction, such as Parkinson's disease
- Helps prevent crooked teeth and tooth decay
- Helps reduce or prevent rheumatoid arthritis

About 80% of Americans are deficient in K2. How much do we need? About 180-200 mg is sufficient per day. [154]

Dr. Kate Rheaume-Bleue, a naturopathic physician, and Dr. Cees Vermeer are 2 experts in this field. I recommend reading their books, or listening to their lectures on YouTube. [154]

K2 is essential for so many things.

These conditions are associated with K2 deficiency.

- osteoporosis
- atherosclerosis
- increased risk of cancer (including breast, prostate, and liver)
- diabetes (helps control insulin production)
- varicose veins
- wrinkles
- dental cavities (takes calcium to the teeth)
- Crohn's disease
- Kidney disease
- narrow, crowded dental arch

I think the most important role of vitamin K2 is its ability to direct calcium where it needs to go. It directs calcium to bones and teeth instead of arteries and other places where it does not belong.

What do we need to help K2 do an effective job with calcium?

First of all, we need to get enough calcium in our diets. Then we need vitamin D3 and magnesium to make the calcium usable. Then it is the job of vitamin K2 to direct the calcium to bones and teeth (or wherever it should be going). Vitamin K2 acts like the usher in a theater. It escorts the calcium to the right spot. Without these four elements, we don't have strong bones and teeth, and we often have calcium in our arteries (hardening of the arteries is calcium), or we have kidney stones, or maybe bone spurs.

K2 is essential to our health in so many ways.

One other vital thing it does is to contribute to the production of **myelin.** Have you heard of the myelin sheath? It is just like the insulation around electrical wires, but it is the protection around the cells in the brain and spinal cord. Inadequate myelin may be what contributes to the occurrence of MS.

Sometimes the thing that gets people's attention is that K2 **reduces wrinkles.**

We used to get lots of vitamin K2. Vitamin K2 comes from eating animals that have been eating what they are supposed to eat (not artificially fed). Cattle are supposed to eat wild grasses. Chickens are supposed to eat such things as seeds, worms, and insects found in fields. However, now that our animals are fed corn and soy-based feed, they (and therefore we) are not getting vitamin K2.

Eggs from pasture-fed hens and gouda and brie cheeses are excellent sources of vitamin K2. Natto (fermented soy) is a popular Japanese food that has K2. [154]

A supplement may also be needed to get enough of these vitamins. If you take supplements, I recommend taking a supplement that contains calcium, magnesium, D3 and K2.

Vitamin D3

Vitamin D is crucial for maintaining our basic health, yet 50% of the general population, and over 95% of seniors are deficient.

Vitamin D is also known as the "sunshine vitamin" because we get vitamin D from exposing our skin to sunshine.

It is probably most famous for being added to milk. This practice helped eliminate rickets.

It is instrumental in turning on about 3,000 genes. We only have about 30,000 total, so vitamin D is crucial for maintaining our basic health.

Almost every cell in our body has a receptor for vitamin D.

The National Health and Nutrition Examination Survey found that 50% of children aged 1-5 and 70% of children between 6 and 11, are deficient in vitamin D.

Seniors are so deficient because they tend to avoid sun exposure, and because they lose their ability to produce vitamin D as they age. [155]

Vitamin D is actually not a vitamin, but a hormone, and something that our body can make if we just get enough sun exposure.

Our best source of vitamin D is to have the sun shine on a minimum 30% of our skin for 10 to 15 minutes per day between 10 and 3. However, many variables may change this number, such as skin color, latitude, season, and clouds in the sky. People with darker skin need more exposure to the sun to get the same amount of vitamin D. Because we have been so afraid of skin cancer, we have been using sunscreen and hats to avoid the sunshine. It is actually **only too much sun exposure that causes cancer.** Moderate exposure actually decreases the chance of getting skin cancer.

What does Vitamin D do?

- Helps eliminate rickets.
- Fights disease, including the flu.
- May reduce risk of multiple scleroses (MS is lower in sunny places).
- Helps with autoimmune diseases, including autoimmune thyroid diseases (Graves' disease and Hashimoto thyroiditis). [156]
- Helps reduce inflammatory bowel disease (lower incidence in sunny environments).
- Reduces heart disease, hypertension, and stroke. In one study, vitamin D deficiency increased the risk of heart attack by 50%. And, if you have a heart attack, and you are vitamin deficient, your risk of dying from that heart attack goes up to almost 100%. [157]
- Improves mood and cognitive disorders.
- Lack of sunlight and low vitamin D contribute to depression.
- Helps regulate other hormones, such as testosterone.
- Has anti-cancer benefits. There may be a protective effect with colon, breast, and prostate cancer. Even skin cancer is reduced with moderate exposure (no burning). The Nurses' Health Studies showed that nurses who had the highest blood levels of 25-hydroxyvitamin D, averaging about 50 ng/ml, reduced their risk of developing breast cancer by as much as 50 percent. [157] Similarly, women who reported having the most sun exposure as

a teenager and young adult had almost a 70 percent reduced risk of developing breast cancer.

- Helps make healthy babies (reducing birth defects) and may reduce the need for a Cesarean.
- It is essential in making calcium usable to the body. If your body doesn't get enough vitamin D, you're at risk of developing bone abnormalities such as soft bones, fragile bones, or osteoporosis. However, remember that you need additional vitamin K2 to take the calcium to the right places.
- Helps reduce obesity.
- Helps with autism, asthma, and tuberculosis.
- Lowers overall mortality.
- Helps reduce incidence of type 1 and type 2 diabetes. It may improve blood sugar and decrease insulin resistance.
- Helps with rheumatoid arthritis (RA).
- Helps reduce hip and knee pain.
- It is crucial for brain development, brain function regulation and a healthy nervous system. Vitamin D deficiency is commonly found in patients with Parkinson's disease, Alzheimer's disease, schizophrenia, depression, anxiety disorders, dementia, and older adults with cognitive decline. Maintaining a healthy level of vitamin D may prevent age-related neurological disorders.

Wow! That is an amazing list. It is very important for everyone to check vitamin D levels, and do what is necessary to increase vitamin D.

The symptoms of a vitamin D deficiency in adults include:

- general tiredness
- aches and pains
- a general sense of not feeling well
- severe bone or muscle pain or weakness that may cause difficulty climbing stairs or getting up from the floor or a low chair, or cause the person to walk with a waddling gait
- problems with kidney function, erectile dysfunction, and sleep apnea.
- stress fractures, especially in the legs, pelvis, and hips. [156]
- mental illness
- obesity

- high blood pressure

However, many people have no symptoms. They may have one of the illnesses mentioned, but neither they nor their doctor attributes it to low vitamin D.

Food sources of Vitamin D

Foods that contain vitamin D are also high in cholesterol. These include:

- **Salmon**
- **Sardines**
- **Egg yolk**
- **Shrimp**

Few foods contain vitamin D naturally. Because of this, some foods are fortified. This means that vitamin D has been added. These include:

- Milk (fortified)
- Yogurt (fortified)
- Cereal (fortified) but not a good choice because of the ingredients
- Orange juice (fortified) but not a good choice because it spikes blood sugar

Blood tests can determine our vitamin D level. What if it is too low? Eat more salmon and eggs. Get more sun exposure without sunscreen. What if it is still too low? Take a supplement. However, supplements are never as good as getting the vitamin naturally.

How strong should the supplement be? We are not sure. The answer varies from 400 IU to 10,000 IU per day, depending on who is doing the research. Vitamin D is fat-soluble, so it needs to be taken with some fat in the diet in order to be used. The fat-soluble vitamins are D, A, E, and K. However, only 20% of our vitamin D is meant to come from our diet. The remaining 80% should come from sun exposure. [156]

The Institute of Medicine (IOM) sets the Recommended Dietary Allowances (RDA). They set the amount needed for most healthy people to avoid diseases. The Endocrine Society sets a level that is optimal rather than the minimum needed, so their numbers are higher. The IOM sets the amount of supplement for 70+ at 800 IU per day. The Endocrine Society sets the amount at 1500 to 2,000 IU per day. Grass Roots Health suggests that adults need about 8,000 IUs per day to achieve a level of 40 ng/ml. (nanograms per milliliter).

Up to 10,000 IU per day can be taken to increase vitamin D levels. However, once levels are up, lowering the dose is recommended.

What should our level of vitamin D be? According to the Endocrine Society, under 30 ng./ml. is insufficient. They say the ideal amount (needed to run your body well) is 40-60 ng./ml. It should not be over 100 ng./ml.

In a large meta-analysis on vitamin D, the lowest mortality was found when levels were over 40 ng/ml.

A study was done on Maasai warriors who were outside every day. This gives us a hint about how much vitamin D our ancestors had. They were found to be around 50 ng./ml.

When it comes to vitamin D, we want to be at an optimum level, not just at the minimum. That may be as high as 50-70 ng./ml. In addition, to treat cancer or heart disease, it may be 70-100 ng./ml. [158]

Unfortunately, as we age, our bodies are less able to absorb vitamin D. Over the age of 70, our vitamin D production may go down as much as 25-30%. [156]

In summary, check your vitamin D levels, eat foods rich in vitamin D, and get lots of sunshine (without burning). To be at optimum health, bring your vitamin D levels up to 50-70 ng./ml.

Magnesium

Magnesium is a mineral we cannot live without. It is involved in about 300 different metabolic reactions in the body. Every cell needs magnesium every second of your life. [44] However, at least 80% of the Westerners are chronically deficient in magnesium. [159]

What foods contain magnesium?

- **nuts**
- **green leafy vegetables**
- **avocados**
- **cacao (chocolate)**
- **raw seeds**
- **squash**

- **fatty fish**
- **fruits and berries**

Most people don't eat enough of these. In addition, modern farming methods deplete the soil of magnesium, and do not add it back. Consequently, most foods that traditionally had magnesium, now don't have much. Therefore, it is important to eat organic foods in order to have the best chance of actually getting magnesium in the foods you eat.

Why do we have low magnesium?

- Our **over-indulgence in eating carbohydrates**. It takes 28 molecules of magnesium to metabolize one molecule of glucose. [160]
- **Magnesium is instrumental in ridding the body of toxins.** We are flooding our bodies with so many toxins in our modern living that our **magnesium cannot keep up.**
- Non-organic farms have so little nutrition in the soil.
- We lose magnesium when we **sweat.**
- **Alcohol** depletes our bodies of magnesium.
- Certain **drugs,** such as statins and fluoride, reduce our magnesium levels. [161]

What happens when we don't get enough magnesium?

- **Magnesium allows our muscles to relax.** Calcium is needed to contract muscles, and magnesium and potassium are needed to relax the muscles. Without sufficient magnesium we have issues with muscles cramping.
- When our muscles can't relax, we can have problems all over our bodies. We get **high blood pressure (from the blood vessels not relaxing), backache, neck pain, muscle spasms around the spline, muscle cramps, irregular heart rhythm, strokes, seizures, migraines, asthma, spastic colon, sudden heart pains, and even sudden cardiac death.** [162]
- Magnesium is instrumental in **brain function** and mood stabilization. Low magnesium is associated with **depression, anxiety, obsessions, hyperactivity, poor memory, vertigo, psychosis, hyperactivity, panic attacks, aggression, and confusion.**

- **Low magnesium may contribute to allergies, hay fever, asthma, and eczema.**
- **Low magnesium will impact the rest of the minerals in the body, such as manganese, copper, zinc, molybdenum, iron, and potassium. It is very difficult to correct these deficiencies without first addressing magnesium levels.** [162] [159]

In addition to eating more foods with magnesium, it may be necessary to take a supplement. Calcium, magnesium, D3 and K2 all work together. It might be a good idea to take all 4 if you decide to take a supplement.

As we age, our bodies are not as good at processing D3 and magnesium. If you are noticing more leg cramps, or are having trouble sleeping, you might consider adding a supplement of magnesium, calcium, D3 and K2.

How much magnesium should we take?

The National Institute of Health recommends 320 mgs. for adult women and 420 mgs. for adult men per day. [163] However, there are many more opinions about how much to take. Dr. Joseph Mercola says, "I believe many may benefit from amounts as high as 1-2 grams per day in divided doses." If you are taking too much magnesium, you will have loose bowel movements. He suggests that this is "disruptive to your microbiome, which would be highly counter-productive." [18]

Other than ingesting magnesium, you can take a bath or soak your feet in Epsom salt (magnesium sulfate). Magnesium can be absorbed through the skin. This should avoid the laxative effect.

If your magnesium levels are adequate, you may need far less vitamin D. Magnesium is needed to activate vitamin D.

(Personal Note)

When I was younger, I noticed that whenever I had a glass of alcohol, I would have leg cramps. However, if I took a magnesium supplement when I drank, the leg cramps did not happen. At age 70, I started taking magnesium daily because I was having leg cramps at night. I also made a point of eating organic foods every day with magnesium. I can remember my mother complaining of leg cramps as she aged.

Now we know. Take magnesium. I also sometimes soak my feet in epson salts for additional magnesium.

Omega 3 vs 6

Because the government subsidizes corn and soybeans, they are very cheap. We feed these cheap products to our animals, and we put them in processed foods. Unfortunately, both corn and soy are very high in omega 6 fatty acids. We need both omega 3 and 6's, but in roughly equal amounts. With our current system of raising animals (feeding them corn and soy) and making processed foods (full of soybean oil and high fructose corn syrup), we are getting up to 18 omega 6's for every omega 3 fatty acid. Our bodies cannot process the omega 3's when they are this out of balance. This is part of why we are so unhealthy.

The easy solution is to not eat the foods artificially high in omega 6's. So, avoid all processed and packaged foods, and eat meat and animal products that are pasture-fed and pasture-finished (not fed soy and corn high in omega 6's).

It is also good to make sure that you are getting enough omega 3's. Wild Alaskan Sockeye salmon is a good source. Many nuts and seeds have high omega 3's.

According to Joseph Hibbeln from the National Institute of Health, consuming too many omega-6 fats and not enough omega-3 fats has led to the following:

- Cardiovascular disease
- Type 2 diabetes
- Obesity
- Metabolic syndrome
- Irritable bowel syndrome
- Inflammatory bowel disease
- Macular degeneration
- Rheumatoid arthritis
- Asthma
- Cancer
- Psychiatric disorders
- Autoimmune diseases

Dr. Hibbeln concludes that the increases in world linoleic acid consumption, primarily from soybean oil (omega-6), and the decrease in consumption of healthy oils (omega-3), has contributed "to increased societal burdens of aggression, depression, and cardiovascular mortality. It's quite likely that most of the diseases of modern civilization, major depression, heart disease, and obesity are linked to the radical and dramatic shift in the composition of the fats in the food supply." [164]

Salt

How much salt should we be eating? There is a range of opinion in the research literature. Let's look at what we know for sure.

Your body needs to be about the same salt concentration as sea water. Our bodies keep our salt balance within a very narrow range. We lose salt when we sweat. That needs to be replaced by consuming more salt. If we eat too much salt, our kidneys filter it out and it leaves our bodies in our urine. We have been told that eating too much salt is very bad for our hearts. However, this may not be true.

Conventional viewpoint on salt from the Center for Disease Control

We have been told that we should limit our salt intake to about 2300 mg per day (about one teaspoon), preferably less. Americans currently consume about 3400 mg per day. [165]

Conventional thinking about salt goes like this:

- When you eat too much salt, your body retains more water to balance the salt content of your body.
- This puts stress on your heart because it has to pump more blood volume.
- This can lead to "developing serious medical conditions, like high blood pressure, heart disease, and stroke." [165]

"Here's the truth: there was never any sound scientific evidence to support this idea." [13]

A low-salt diet

What actually happens when we reduce sodium intake? These are some **health risks of low sodium intake:** [13]

- Increased heart rate
- Compromised kidney function
- Hypothyroidism
- Higher triglyceride, cholesterol, and insulin levels
- Insulin resistance
- Obesity
- Type 2 diabetes

Let's look at just one of these: insulin resistance.

When we are low in sodium, **"One of the body's defense mechanisms is to increase insulin levels, because insulin helps the kidneys retain more sodium."** [13]

Steady high insulin levels (leading to insulin resistance) may be the underlying cause of many of our diseases. **The last thing we need is to be increasing our insulin levels through lack of salt in our diets.**

Are you eating low salt?

Many people think that if they don't add salt to their food, they are eating a low-salt diet. This is not true (unless you cook your own food). **The "majority of the sodium Americans consume --more than 70% -- is found in processed food and restaurant meals."** [165]

Standard view of sodium:

Both sodium and potassium affect blood pressure. According to the CDC, "People who reduce sodium, who increase potassium, or who do both benefit from having lower blood pressure and reducing their risk for other serious health problems." [165]

Many organizations, including the American Heart Association, the American Medical Association and the American Public Health Association, support reducing dietary sodium intake. The 2010 Dietary Guidelines for Americans suggests that we "reduce daily sodium intake to less than 2,300 milligrams (mg) and further reduce intake to 1,500 mg among persons who are 51 years of age and older and those of any age who are African American or have hypertension, diabetes, or chronic kidney disease."

Other viewpoints: Maybe limiting salt is not a good idea

As I did research for this book, I discovered that the opinions about salt range from *radically reducing salt intake*, to eating *more* salt in order to *reduce* heart attacks.

Mark Hyman, M.D., author of *Food What the Heck Should I Eat?* [21] **suggests these things:**

The type of salt we eat matters:

Regular table salt, and the salt in most packaged foods, is not good for you. It is a manufactured chemical (sodium chloride), to be avoided.

Instead, use natural salts, such as pink Himalayan sea salt. They contain natural minerals that our bodies need.

Do not use iodized salt.

He says that reducing salt may not be of value:

If you are diagnosed with high blood pressure, you will probably be told to reduce your salt intake. This may not be good advice.

The research doesn't show much benefit to restricting salt. [21]

How much salt does he recommend?

He, like the CDC, recommends about 2300 milligrams per day of salt.

Instead of adding salt, he recommends:

Eating foods rich in natural sodium to meet your salt requirements.

Like the CDC, he stresses the importance of potassium.

Be sure to get enough potassium in your diet. Potassium and sodium need to be in balance. [21]

What foods are rich in sodium?

Meat	Celery	Beans
Beets	Chard	
Carrots	Seaweed	

What foods are rich in potassium?

Papayas	Squash	Avocados

Broccoli	Spinach	Melons
Bananas	Raisins	Pears
Potatoes	Mango	
Mushrooms	Oranges	

We usually don't think of table salt as a processed food, but it is, and should be avoided. "The highly refined salt that food manufacturers add to processed and packaged foods is killing us." [21]

Other opinions:

Does high salt intake really raise blood pressure?

- 80% of people with normal blood pressure (less than 120/80 mm/Hg) have no reaction to eating more salt.
- Among those with prehypertension, roughly 75% have no reaction.
- Even among those with full-blown hypertension, about 55% have no reaction. [166]

So, consuming salt has absolutely no impact on raising blood pressure in most people. That is clearly not what we have been told.

Q: Even in those with hypertension (blood pressure of 140/90 mmHg or higher) how much does blood pressure go down if we restrict salt?
A: 3.6 mmHg on systolic blood pressure, and 1.6 mmHg on diastolic blood pressure. [167] That is a very small change. That is like going from 140/90 to 137.5/88.4. Not much.

Q: What about those with normal blood pressure (less than 120/80)?
A: Reducing your salt intake to "around 2,300 milligrams per day (1 teaspoon of salt) may only lower your blood pressure by a meager 0.8/.0.2mmHg." [167] [13]

Q: What causes high blood pressure if it is not salt?
A: All sugar, but fructose in particular.
Only 5% of adults had high blood pressure in 1900. Now 31% of

adults have high blood pressure. [60]

Q: Why has blood pressure increased so much since 1900?
A: Fructose has been added to so many of our processed foods. [60]

High fructose corn syrup (HFCS) has "increased 10,673 percent between 1970 and 2005, according to the USDA. It now makes up the **number one source of calories in America**." [60]

We now consume 70 grams of fructose every day. In 1900, we only ate 15 grams of fructose, and that was mostly fruit.

In addition to limiting fructose, avoid or limit all foods that spike blood sugar, including whole wheat, breads, pasta, rice, cereal, and potatoes.

The advice to severely restrict salt intake (below 1500 mg. per day) may actually lead to more heart problems.

In summary, to lower blood pressure

- **Limit all sugars, but fructose in particular**
- **Limit anything with a high glycemic index**
- **Eat more potassium**
- **Eat natural salt, such as Himalayan salt**
- **Avoid table salt and salt in processed foods**

Our bodies need to stay at a certain level of salt. No too much and not too little. If we eat too much, and if we have healthy kidneys, our kidneys filter out the extra salt and it leaves our bodies in our urine. But if we have too little salt, our bodies cannot make it. We have to eat it. In addition, the kidneys increase insulin as part of the process of conserving our salt. We don't need more insulin. Consequently, the danger really is in not getting enough salt, not too much salt.

It seems strange to say this after so many years of being told to lower our salt intake, but, if your kidneys work well, [168] **make sure you are getting enough healthy salt in your diet.**

Take Away

- Vitamins K2, D3, and magnesium are so important that we should make sure we are getting enough of these every day. Sadly, most Americans are deficient in all three.
- It is also important the get enough Omega 3 fatty acids. We are not only not eating enough omega 3's, but we are eating way too many omega 6's. So, add more omega 3's, and also cut back on omega 6's. We need both but in roughly the same amount.
- Salt is very controversial. The research says that if your kidneys are functioning well, perhaps you should be adding more healthy salt to your diet to avoid increased insulin.

Chapter 9

The Ecosystem In
Us And Around Us

A well-functioning gut with healthy gut flora holds the roots of our health. And, just as a tree with sick roots is not going to thrive, the rest of the body cannot thrive without a well-functioning digestive system.

--Dr. Natasha Campbell-McBride [138]

How we digest food, or the "food tube"

Think about digestion as your food going in your mouth and traveling through a tube and coming out the other end. It gets broken down various ways, leaves the tube at various points, then travels through your bloodstream in order to feed all the cells of your body. It is very important that all of this goes well if you want all of the cells of your body to be adequately nourished.

Also, your body is constantly making new cells to replace older cells. You need to give your body the basic building blocks of each cell in order for them to be made correctly. Let's go through how this works.

Digestion begins in the mouth

Your teeth chew the food into smaller pieces. You need to have good teeth and gums. Chronic inflammation in the gums or decay in the teeth can profoundly affect your overall health. In your mouth, the food gets mixed with saliva. Saliva has important ingredients that help in the digestive process. It's important that food spends adequate time in the mouth for these things to happen. That is why you are supposed to thoroughly chew each bite of food. [169]

Drinking liquids with your food may not be a good idea. Liquids dilute the saliva, stomach acid, and other digestive juices along the way. Consider drinking liquids a few hours before eating, and stop drinking 30 minutes before eating. Then wait 2 hours after eating before resuming drinking again. A few sips of liquid with a meal are OK. [169]

In addition, drinking our meals (protein shakes, etc.) interferes with the digestion that should start in the mouth.

Digestion of carbohydrates begins here.

Both chewing and salivating signal the rest of the digestive system that food is coming.

Q: What is the average amount of "chews" Americans do before swallowing? [168]

A: Four and a half! Not nearly enough. We should be chewing our food until it is a liquid. Digestive problems can be created by simply not chewing enough.

Mouth and Teeth

Did you know that your oral health offers clues about your overall health — or that problems in your mouth can affect the rest of your body?

--Mayo Clinic [170]

Before we continue with digestion, let's look at oral health more closely.

How is your oral health connected to your overall health?

"The Oral Microbiome is a whole ecosystem unto itself, which when in balance gives us health, and when it is out of balance, gives us

disease."

--Bonnie Feldman, DDS [171]

Bacteria that cause diseases enter your body primarily through the mouth, and secondarily through the nose and eyes, and occasionally through a cut in the skin.

The balance of bacteria in the mouth is important for your health. We used to think that all bacteria in the mouth are bad. That is why anti-bacterial mouthwashes became so popular. However, we have discovered that most bacteria in the mouth are good for us, and that it is important to keep a healthy balance of microbiome in the mouth, just as it is important to maintain a healthy gut microbiome.

Bacteria have been evolving for millions of years. We swallow 150 billion to a trillion bacteria each day. [172] These bacteria have a huge impact on our general health. Oral bacteria have been linked to heart disease, diabetes, Alzheimer's, gut health, aching joints, and more. It is extremely important to keep your oral bacteria in a healthy balance.

How to we keep our mouths healthy?

Saliva

Having a healthy amount of saliva is essential for oral health. In fact, **it is lack of saliva that may be the primary cause of tooth decay.** [172] Eating sugar is still a problem, but it may not be as much of a problem as a dry mouth. Saliva helps to neutralize acids produced by bacteria in the mouth. It also helps wash away food.

Why do people have dry mouth?

- Certain medications can reduce saliva. Some medications that may reduce saliva are decongestants, antihistamines, painkillers, diuretics and antidepressants.
- Breathing through the mouth, especially at night, can cause many problems with the teeth and gums.
- Not being adequately hydrated.

Brush and floss

This helps reduce tooth decay and gum disease. Gum inflammation is associated with other diseases in the body. If gums are inflamed, the bacteria can travel directly into your bloodstream to other parts of your body, such as your heart, and cause problems.

Get a new tooth brush if yours looks worn.

What other conditions can be linked to oral health?

- Pregnancy and birth complications
- Pneumonia
- Diabetes
- Osteoporosis
- Alzheimer's disease
- Eating disorders
- Rheumatoid arthritis
- Certain cancers

These conditions are associated with poor oral health. That doesn't mean that there is a causal relationship. For example, perhaps tooth problems and osteoporosis are both caused by lack of vitamin K2. Or perhaps all of these problems are caused by eating too much sugar. In other words, we find that poor oral health goes hand in hand with many other diseases. [170]

How can I protect my oral health?

Practice good oral hygiene daily

- Brush your teeth at least twice a day with a soft-bristled brush.
- Floss daily.
- Eat a healthy diet
- Replace your toothbrush every three months or sooner if bristles are worn.
- Schedule regular dental checkups and cleanings, perhaps every 3-6 months.
- Stop smoking and/or chewing tobacco. [170]

Mercury in fillings

- "Silver" fillings are usually 52% mercury. Over time, mercury leaks into our bodies. It is anti-microbial, so it may be killing some of our gut microbiome. In addition, it goes into the organs of our bodies, in particular our brains. Mercury poisoning has been linked to fatigue, anxiety and insomnia.

- Some people genetically have a difficulty eliminating heavy metals. Others get rid of them just fine, so not everyone will have this problem. [172]

Back to digestion:

Esophagus

The esophagus leads from the throat to the stomach. The stomach produces very caustic acids to aid in digestion. There is a muscle at the top of the stomach that keeps the food and stomach acids from going back into the esophagus. However, sometimes these stomach acids do leak back into the esophagus. This is called heartburn or GERD (Gastroesophageal reflux disease). This can be very painful. What you eat is a major factor in creating this problem.

How to prevent this? Eat real food. After eating it is best to not lie down for a period of time in order to give your stomach a chance to do its job and to pass the food along (usually a minimum of 2 hours).

Stomach

The stomach adds acid and enzymes to the food and the stomach muscles churn the food. The stomach is very acidic. This kills almost all bacteria. Some few survive the stomach acid. Taking antacids is a problem because it increases the PH of the stomach, allowing too many bacteria to survive.

Digestion of protein begins here.

By the time the food leaves the stomach, it is a liquid or paste.

If you eat too frequently, the stomach does not have enough time to thoroughly digest each meal.

The stomach lining is protected by a thick layer of mucous. Otherwise, the stomach lining would be damaged by the stomach acid.

Food spends 2-4 hours in the stomach.

Small intestine

The small intestine is about 20 feet long. The pancreas, liver, and gall bladder add more digestive juices to the food.

The food is a liquid at this stage. It is here that much of the food moves out of the intestines and into the bloodstream to go to the cells. Food is here about 3-5 hours.

Liver

The liver is one of our most important organs. It is about the size of a football, and is protected by the ribcage. We can't live without it. The liver performs more than 500 vital functions. [173] Some of the liver's jobs are to:

- **Filter blood.** As food is digested and goes into the blood, it first passes through the liver. It filters 30% of your blood every minute. The liver maintains healthy levels of many things in your body, such as glucose and cholesterol.
- **Remove toxins.** It metabolizes drugs and alcohol and removes damaged cells and anything it perceives as toxic.
- **Add bile to the food to help with digestion.** Although bile is made in the liver, it is stored in the gallbladder. Bile is primarily used to digest fat.
- **Make proteins**. We need a constant supply of new proteins. The liver makes these proteins. It makes many proteins that are important for blood clotting.
- **Break down fat and make cholesterol**. Most of our cholesterol is made by the liver. A small amount, maybe 15-20%, comes from our food.
- **Convert glucose to glycogen**. The liver then stores glycogen until it is ready for use, then it converts it back to glucose.
- **Convert amino acids into glucose.**
- **Store vitamins and minerals** until your body needs them.
- **Create immune factors** that are necessary in fighting infection.
- **Store important nutrients for immediate use.** [173]

When the liver is damaged, these things can't happen. If the liver is damaged enough, and toxins do not get removed from the blood, it can lead to brain damage and coma, and eventually death.

Fortunately, the liver can regenerate. If there is enough healthy liver left, it can grow the rest back. It is a very resilient organ, but it has its limits.

Taking good care of the liver is primarily about avoiding toxins such as alcohol, cleaning products, and any medicines, even things like

OTC pain killers or cough medicine.

Appendix

The appendix is located at the junction of the small and large intestines. We used to think that it did not serve any purpose, but we now believe that it serves as a place for the "gut bacteria" to be stored in case we need to eliminate everything in the "food tube" (Bollinger, Barbas, Bush, Lin, & Parker, 2007). If you eat something that your body determines is toxic, your body will empty out the "food tube" (vomiting and diarrhea). This includes all of the beneficial bacteria. The appendix stores these beneficial bacteria, and repopulates the large intestine. These intestinal bacteria must be very important to have a structure devoted to making sure we maintain the huge range of bacteria we need to stay healthy. [174]

Large intestine

The large intestine is 5 to 6 feet long. We used to think that this is where food gets ready for elimination and not much else. It does take the liquid out of the food and leaves it in a firmer state for elimination. However, we have come to realize that the **3 pounds of bacteria that live here are crucial to:**

- **Digesting our food**
- **Boosting our immune system**
- **Creating much of the nutrition that we need to function**
- **Sending information through our nervous system to our brain**
- **Turning many of our genes on and off**

Food is here 4 to 72 hours, averaging about 36 hours.

Rectum and Anus

The rectum is about 8 inches long and connects the large intestine to the anus. From the rectum, the food is eliminated. By looking at what comes out, it is possible to tell how healthy you are. If you are eating healthy food, and drinking enough water, you should be having easy daily eliminations, with no diarrhea.

All of the parts of the digestive system need to be in good working order in order for us to stay healthy.

What should our poop look like?

- Ideally, it should be brown and look like a log or a snake.
- Any other color besides brown means there is a problem (yellow, green, red, etc.).
- If it is dark and looks like hard nuts or pebbles, and is hard to pass, this is a sign that we are dehydrated, or that we need to speed up the time it takes to go through our bodies (transit time). It could also mean there are gall bladder issues.
- Diarrhea or loose stools means that our bodies are trying to get rid of toxic foods, or we have a food intolerance, or perhaps a stomach bug. Alcohol, caffeine and stress can also cause diarrhea.
- If you can identify what you just ate, you may have insufficient enzymes, aren't chewing enough, or food is going through you too quickly (except for corn, which does go through somewhat unchanged). [168]
- Dairy, gluten, processed soy, sugar, and shellfish can cause digestive disorders and change our poop.
- Poop can be green or red if you have eaten lots of green or red foods, but they should not be odd colors normally.
- Most mammals, regardless of their size, produce bowel movements in about 12 seconds. If you are taking a long time or are straining, this is a sign that something is wrong. [175]

Poop should come out easily. Pooping 1-3 times a day is normal. Pooping less often than every 3 days is constipation. If you are having issues, try eating more fiber (fruits and vegetables), drinking more water, managing stress, sleeping more, and exercising more. [176]

When does it go from the "food tube" into our bodies?

In a way, the food in the "food tube" is not really a part of our bodies. Only when the small particles of food leave the tube do they really become "us".

Where does this food leave the "food tube" and become nutrition for our cells?

Alcohol

About 20% of alcohol is absorbed by the stomach into the bloodstream, and the other 80% is absorbed by the small intestine. This takes from a few minutes to 2 hours to be fully absorbed. The body considers alcohol a poison, and the liver is responsible for taking poisons out of the bloodstream. That is why drinking too much alcohol puts such a strain on your liver.

Sugar

Sugar is very quickly digested and sent into the bloodstream. If a sugary food is eaten by itself, people will experience a "sugar rush". This lasts typically from 15 to 40 minutes, followed by an energy crash. The more processed the food (like white flour), the more it is digested quickly, like sugar.

How long does it take from eating to elimination?

In general, it takes about 30-50 hours to digest a meal. It depends on what you have eaten, and your gender. Women take an average of 47 hours to digest a meal, whereas men take only 33 hours. One way to test your transit time is to eat corn or beets. You can see the corn, and the beets will be red.

Meat takes about 2 days to digest. That is why it is said that meat may contribute to having colon cancer. It sits longer in the colon. Fruits and vegetables take about a day. Sugar and candy are digested within hours. [176]

It only takes 6-8 hours for the food to pass through the stomach and small intestine. Most of the time is spent in the large intestine.

Gut bacteria

All diseases begin in the gut.
--Hippocrates (460-370 BC)

Hippocrates is the father of modern medicine. He got it right so many years ago! Our digestive system, and more specifically, our gut bacteria, hold the key to our health.

Vegetables contain large amounts of fiber that we cannot digest. However, our gut bacteria depend on this fiber.

You will grow the kind of bacteria you need to digest the foods you eat. If you eat sugary foods, that bacteria will thrive. If you eat lots of broccoli or beans, then those bacteria will thrive.

Some researchers believe that the vagus nerve, which travels from our brain to our intestines has a 2-way signaling system. Not only does the brain tell the digestive system what to do (stop digestion because we are running), but signals go from the digestive system to the brain.

If we are used to eating sugary foods, and we have lots of bacteria that digest sugary foods, those bacteria send signals to our brain, and we crave sugary foods. However, when we switch to eating vegetables, we develop more bacteria that digest vegetables, and we gradually want to eat more vegetables. The bacteria, to some extent, dictate what we want to eat.

Interesting fact: People who eliminate added sugars often report losing their sugar cravings after they get used to eating healthy foods. This could take only a week, but it may take 2-3 weeks. [96] Our intestinal bacteria change very quickly.

Question: In all of the cells that live in our bodies, how much of the DNA is human?
A: In addition to human DNA, we also have living in and on us:

Bacteria	Yeast
Viruses	Parasites

Only 10-50% is human. Most of the other 50-90% is bacteria, primarily in our gut.

Why do "gut bacteria" matter?

Healthy gut bacteria provide the following:

- **boost your immune system (About 80% of our immune system is located in our gut)**
- **help increase energy**
- **improve your sleep**
- **balance stress levels**
- **lower your risk for cancer and other diseases**
- **help you lose weight** [177]

It is vital to our health that we have a good range of healthy gut bacteria.

About 3 pounds of bacteria live in our intestines (our brains are about 3 pounds). The "gut bacteria" is sometimes called our "second brain" because it controls so many of our processes.

Now, let's look at the bacteria all around us – bacteria we need in order to be healthy.

Where do we get his range of gut bacteria?

Right before birth, the mother's bacteria move from her anus to her vagina. As the infant passes through the birth canal, the newborn is covered with the mom's gut bacteria. In addition, breast milk continues to deliver bacteria to her baby. Breast milk also has some sugars in it that the baby cannot digest. These sugars are there to feed the new bacteria in the gut.

The child also gets bacteria from the environment. If there is a dog in the home, children have a larger range of biodiversity in their gut. Interestingly, a cat in the home doesn't seem to make any difference.

The child also gets it from being in the natural environment. Bacteria come from dirt, the park, the beach, the forest, etc.

Eventually, the child gets more gut bacteria from food. At about 2 years old, the child should have a full range of gut bacteria.

Are bacteria friend or foe?

We have been taught that bacteria and viruses are the enemy and are to be avoided or killed whenever possible.

Some few viruses and bacteria are the enemy, such as the flu, colds, and diseases like small pox, the plague, etc.

However, there are 100 trillion bacteria, fungus, parasites and mold living in and on us all of the time. Without them, we would die. We have a symbiotic relationship with them. We need them, and they need us.

Some examples of the critters living in and on us:

Of course, there are our **gut bacteria**.

Mites live on our eyelashes and eyebrows. They burrow into our hair follicles.

There are two different kinds of mites on our faces. They live in our oil glands. They come out at night to mate, then go back in in the morning. Yuck!

There is a **fungus that lives on our feet** (that distinctive "old sock" smell).

There is a type of **bacteria that lives in our armpit**. Have you noticed that many animals sniff each other's posteriors? You can see this most noticeably in dogs. From the odor, they can tell such things as:

- The sex of the animal
- If female, where she is in her cycle (Is it time to mate?)
- How closely related they are (Is she my cousin?) [178]

When humans started walking upright, this scent was moved to the armpit for humans. We are not consciously aware of these messages, but our behavior is directed by many of these processes that our conscious mind does not know are happening.

Most of our body odors are not coming from us. We have almost no odor. The odors are from the particular bacteria and fungi that grow on us.

Our skin is covered with a coat of various kinds of bacteria. These are our first line of defense. If an unwanted bacterium tries to get a foothold in us, the healthy bacteria don't let it in.

Joke:

Some disease bacteria walk into a bar and say "give us a drink".

The bartender says, "We don't serve your type here".

The disease bacteria say, "You are not much of a host".

Taken loosely from the movie *Life on Us: A Microscopic Safari*. [179]

Bathing gets rid of most bacteria on our skin. Yes, it feels good, we smell better, but it also removes our protective bacteria. Fortunately, they quickly repopulate on our skin, but it leaves an opening for undesirable bacteria to get a foothold and thrive.

Gut microbes have been found to influence a number of diseases, obesity, mental health and behavior, and even gene expression in the areas of learning, memory, and motor control.

How do we increase our healthy gut bacteria?

- Eat fermented foods.
- Eliminate sugar from our diets
- Eliminate processed and packaged foods

How do we damage our healthy gut bacteria?

- Taking antibiotics (to be used only when absolutely necessary)
- Drinking chlorinated water
- Using antibacterial soap
- Eating conventionally raised meats (due to their antibiotic exposure and residue of glyphosate)
- Eating conventionally raised fruits and vegetables (due to their residue of glyphosate)

Fecal transplants

Sometimes people have gut bacteria that are severely out of balance. There are too many unhealthy bacteria and not enough healthy ones. These cases are often successfully treated with antibiotics. However, sometimes the antibiotics kill too many of the healthy gut bacteria so that the patient cannot recover.

Fecal transplant to the rescue!

The most successfully treated cases involve patients who have C. difficile, or C. diff. This is a disease that involves a severe intestinal infection that is not responding to antibiotics.

A fecal transplant consists of taking fecal matter (poop) from a healthy donor and putting it into someone who needs better intestinal bacteria.

Fecal transplants have been 85-90% successful in restoring the gut's healthy bacterial balance.

Fecal transplants may also be useful on people with:

- Ulcerative colitis
- Crohn's disease
- Cirrhosis
- Multiple sclerosis
- Depression
- Obesity
- Food allergies
- Diabetes

It has been shown to have a profound effect on obese rats (obese rats receiving fecal transplants from thin rats). This indicates that some part of obesity may be due to gut bacteria.

Warning: Do this only with a doctor's help. Do not do this on your own. The donor has to be carefully screened.

Gut health and soil health --- the role of pesticides and herbicides

We are only as healthy as the soil that grew our food. Pesticides and herbicides kill healthy organisms in the soil, so our food has very little nutrition, unless it is organically grown. Fertilizer adds only a few micronutrients (nitrogen, potassium, and phosphorus).

When our food grows, it absorbs the micronutrients in the soil. It can only get the micronutrients that are there. When we kill the organisms in the soil, they cannot make the micronutrients we need.

We are poisoning our food. When we eat food that has been sprayed with poison, we usually can't wash the poison off. It is inside the plant. We eat the poison. The poison kills our "gut bacteria" just as it kills the bacteria in the soil.

There are 3 levels to the damage done by herbicides and pesticides (primarily glyphosate – the chemical in Roundup).

- They **kill the biodiversity of our gut bacteria** which are instrumental in being able to digest food.
- The poisons that we put on our food **break down the thin barrier lining of our digestive wall** which allows the poisons in our digestive system to leak into our bodies. This is called **"leaky gut"**.
- These poisons actually break down all of the walls all over our body. **Our brains are experiencing leaking through the capillary walls.** [180]

A plant's ecosystem

We tend to lose sight of the fact that we are part of an ecosystem. We depend on the life around us to keep us healthy. We depend on the food, the air, the soil, and all aspects of our environment.

We are only as healthy as the food we eat. The food we eat is only as healthy as the food it ate. We know animals eat food, and their health depends on what they eat. In addition, our vegetables also live in a very complicated ecosystem. That ecosystem determines how healthy the vegetables are. We cannot artificially change the ecosystems of our food sources and expect that we will get healthy food from these artificial environments.

Dirt plus organic matter equals healthy living soil.

What kind of organic matter?

In one teaspoon of healthy living soil, how many of each of these would you find?

- **Bacteria,** one-celled organisms that are decomposers
- **Fungi,** grows as long threads. Most fungi are decomposers that break down more complex carbons. Mycorrhizal fungi assist 90% of plants in obtaining nutrients.
- **Actinomycetes, a large group of bacteria.** The "earthy" smell of soil comes from these.
- **Protozoa,** large one-celled organisms that help in recycling by feeding on bacteria
- **Nematodes**, non-segmented worms

How many in only one teaspoon?

- Bacteria, 1 billion!!
- Fungi, 100 yards
- Actinomycetes, 1,000
- Protozoa, 2,000
- Nematodes, 100 [181]

The plant miraculously uses photosynthesis to turn the energy in sunshine into plant matter. Plants share their food with the microbes in the soil. Bacteria protect the roots, and the fungi share minerals and other nutrients with the plant roots. Everything eats and is eaten.

This system is true of organic soil. However, when **pesticides and herbicides are used on the plants, the soil becomes largely dead. We no longer see this rich abundance in the ecosystem, and therefore our food lacks nutrition. This is why it is so important to eat organic food whenever possible.** However, if you feel that organic is too expensive or you do not have adequate access to organic food, it is still better to eat conventional produce than no produce at all.

Poison in our food and GMO's

Glyphosate is a poison which is the main ingredient in Roundup. Glyphosate is the most-used agricultural chemical ever! Americans have applied 1.8 million tons of glyphosate since 1974. Worldwide, 9.4 million tons of the chemical have been used. In addition, it is becoming more and more of a problem. In 1987, 11 million pounds of the chemical were used on U.S. farms. That sounds like a lot, but now nearly 300 million pounds of glyphosate are applied each year. And it is only getting worse as weeds become more resistant to the poison.

In March of 2015, the World Health Organization's International Agency for Research on Cancer unanimously determined that glyphosate is "probably carcinogenic to humans". A carcinogen is a substance known to cause cancer.

In addition, glyphosate is an endocrine disruptor. It interferes with the production and function of hormones. It is unclear how much impact glyphosate has had on the cancer rate increasing. [182]

Not surprisingly, Monsanto (the company that makes glyphosate), maintains that it is safe for human consumption.

Exactly what is a Genetically Modified Organism or "GMO" and how is that related to poison sprayed on our food?

GMO stands for "genetically modified organism". There are many forms of genetically modified plants and animals, but the specific type of GMO of interest here relates to changes made to our food.

The first commercially useful genetically modified food was a tomato that had a longer "shelf life" because it took longer to ripen. Many of us can remember when tomatoes would go bad very quickly, but they also had much more flavor. Now they sit on the counter for weeks without going bad. As the genetic modifications to the tomato changed the shelf life, the taste also changed. Did it also change the nutritional value? We don't know. How does this new tomato interact with our bodies? We have no idea.

Monsanto is the company famous for producing Genetically Modified foods. They start with a traditional plant, such as a soybean, and splice a piece of the gene of another plant or animal into the soybean DNA structure. Monsanto does this with vegetables to make them "roundup ready". This means that Monsanto can put large amounts of poison on the plant, and that plant won't die. The weeds around the plant should die, but the specific genetically modified plant shouldn't die.

Also, more and more poison is needed to do the same job because the weeds become resistant to the poison. This is not sustainable.

Most genetically modified crops are changed so that they will have increased resistance to herbicides.

In 2016, salmon were genetically modified with growth hormones so that they would grow faster.

What are we even eating if we consume a GMO food? We don't really know!

Monsanto is the company that has brought us many of the most toxic products over the last 50 years, including Agent Orange, PCB's and dioxin, DDT, saccharin, and aspartame. [46]

What is the poison doing to us?

Why are we spraying food with poison? Yes, to kill the weeds, but what is it doing to us? Keep in mind that of all of the DNA in us and on us, most of it is not human DNA. For example, what is it doing to our gut microbiome? We need the bacteria in our gut to be healthy, so that we can stay healthy.

Sixty-four countries require **GMO labeling**, including the European Union (where GMOs are banned), Japan, Australia, Brazil, Russia, and even China, **but not the United States.** [46]

These are the top GMO foods:

- Soy.
- Corn, including high fructose corn syrup, corn oil, and corn syrup.
- Sugar Beets. Most sugar is made from this.
- Canola oil
- Cotton, including cottonseed oil
- Alfalfa
- Zucchini and yellow squash
- Papaya

Eat these at your peril.

Bottom line: Almost all the little creatures in us and on us are our friends. We need them to survive. We are all part of the life around us. Be grateful they are there. Treat them well. This goes for our little personal ecosystem and for the larger ecosystem of our environment.

Processed Foods vs. Organic

Processed foods

We are meant to eat foods just as they come to us in nature. Nature provides packages of nutrition. If we eat food exactly as it comes, we get everything we need to digest and use that particular food. For example, if we eat an orange, it comes with enough fiber to slow down digestion, so the sugar in the orange does not spike our blood sugar so much.

However, natural food spoils quickly. In addition, most foods are only ripe and ready to eat at certain times of the year. To deal with these two issues, we have developed processed foods. They last for a long time on the grocery shelf, or in our kitchens. We can eat them all year, no matter what the season.

Sugar and white flour are two processed foods that we have been eating for centuries.

Wheat, in particular, has been hugely advantageous in human evolution. This has allowed humans to have a steady supply of food that can be easily stored.

What exactly is processed food, and why is it so bad for us? As we process food, it loses not only its nutritional value, but also its flavor. To give processed food enough flavor, and to keep it longer on the shelf, more chemicals are added.

In summary, processed foods are easy to store, easy to eat, available in abundance, and are a source of cheap calories, but have very little nutrition, and may have poisons in the form of herbicides and pesticides and added chemicals.

Organic foods

In order to be labeled organic, farmers cannot use:

- Pesticides
- Synthetic fertilizers
- Sewage sludge
- Genetically modified organisms (GMO)
- Ionizing radiation
- Antibiotics
- Growth hormones

In summary, why eat organic rather than conventionally grown food?

- Organic food has more nutrition.
- Most organic food tastes better.
- Approximately 50-70% of our drinking water has pesticides in it. Supporting organic growers means safer drinking water.
- Some pesticides, called organophosphates, were originally developed as toxic nerve gas. These have been adapted to kill pests on foods. Exposure to these pesticides may lead to nerve damage in humans.
- Children may be more at risk because their brains and bodies are

forming.

- Eighteen per cent of all genetically modified seeds make their own pesticides. They become part of the plant, and then part of you, if you eat them.
- Pesticides damage wildlife and wildlife habitat.
- Pesticides may be contributing to the increase in cancer.

Quiz: Why are conventionally grown fruits and vegetables not as healthy as organic?

Answer:

- **You are eating the poison that is sprayed on fruits and vegetables and that poison kills our gut bacteria.**
- **The poison kills the healthy bacteria in the soil so the soil has very little nutrition to give to the plant.**

$$\boxed{\text{Take Away}}$$

- We have a very complicated ecosystem on us and in us. We have bacteria on our skin, we have special bacteria in our mouths, and we have 3 pounds of bacteria in our large intestine. These are all vital to our health. Instead of seeing bacteria and viruses as our enemy, we should be doing things to support their health. Our lives depend on these little critters.
- In addition, we have a very complicated ecosystem all around us. Healthy food depends on these little organisms. Our health depends on this healthy food.
- We should be doing our best to eliminate poisons and chemicals in and on our food. We should not eat meat that has been grown with added hormones or antibiotics. We should be avoiding all GMO foods. Eat organic whenever possible.

Chapter 10

Our Ancestors and Our Children

What did your ancestors eat?

We have been evolving for millions of years. The human species has been around for 100,000 to 400,000 years (depending on how we define human). It has only been over the last few hundred years that we have been mixing our genes together from around the world. Up until a few hundred years ago, we didn't travel very far from our place of birth. There were invasions from other regions, such as the Romans, Alexander the Great, or Napoleon, but when you consider the entire planet, these were fairly local invasions.

My ancestors were from northern Europe. I had my ancestry done (23 and Me). I am from the British Isles, Scandinavia, and Northern Europe. Traditionally, what did these folks eat? Up until 10,000 years ago, when they were primarily hunter/gatherers, they probably ate meat, fish, and root vegetables all winter. Then during the warm months, they added a good range of vegetables and fruits when they were available. They might have occasionally eaten some honey.

From 400,000 years ago up until about 40,000 years ago, the Neanderthals populated Europe. There were other species of humanoids living in other regions of the world. The first wave of genetically modern humans to leave Africa probably took place about 100,000 years ago. They interbred with the Neanderthals (and the Neanderthals disappeared as a separate species), and the humans took over Europe as the dominant species. So, probably **humans have been living in and developing their particular compatibility with the plants and animals in each area for up to 100,000 years ago in Europe.**

About 10,000 years ago, Europe began the domestication of animals, and growing crops for food. They domesticated cows for dairy, such as milk and cheese. Food was abundant during the warm months, so they ate a large variety of fruits and vegetables, but what did they eat all winter? They ate what they had eaten as hunter/gatherers: meat and root vegetables. But now, in addition, they had milk, milk products, and meat from their domesticated animals, and whatever they could store from their crops. What was that? Probably grains. You might imagine they also had potatoes, but potatoes came from South America just a few hundred years ago.

What was the impact of farming?

Beginning 10,000 years ago, we became smaller and less healthy, with smaller brains, probably because of the grains we began eating, combined with the close association with animals and their diseases.

However, having control of our food supply gave us the ability to feed large numbers of people easily. This was the beginning of towns, and then cities. It also gave people more leisure time. **This steady food supply made advanced civilization possible.**

What were the variety of diets?

What exactly were these diets around the world? There is no diet that fits everyone. It varied radically from place to place.

On one extreme, we have the Inuit who eat primarily meat, fish, and fat.

Then we have the Okinawans who eat almost exclusively a plant-based diet, mostly sweet potatoes. [102]

Twenty per cent of our calories go to feeding our brains. An ape's brain only requires eight per cent of its calories. It is believed that we were able to develop our large brains when we switched from being primarily vegetarians (like apes) to eating meat.

After studying the diets of living hunter-gatherers, Loren Cordain wrote the book, *The Paleo Diet: Lose Weight and Get Healthy by Eating the Foods You were Designed to Eat*. He concluded that 73% of primitive societies got half of their calories from meat. **He recommended that we eat meat and fish, but not dairy, grains, or beans (all introduced after agriculture began, about 10,000 years ago).** Interestingly, dairy, grains and beans are the foods that many people have negative reactions to. **He suggests that we will avoid all of the diseases of civilization such as heart disease, cancer, high blood pressure, diabetes, and even acne, if we stick to this diet.**

Anthropologists debate whether agriculture was good for human health. We began to have cavities and other dental problems for the first time. We got shorter. Our diets were less nutritionally diverse.

What were our first agricultural crops? They were thought to be wheat, sorghum, barley, corn and rice. From eating largely the same foods every day, we start seeing nutritional deficiency.

However, our DNA continues to evolve.

Over the last 10,000 years, our teeth, jaws, and faces have gotten smaller.

Those areas that domesticated cattle developed lactose tolerance. Lactose is a form of sugar that is in milk. Areas that did not have cattle remained lactose intolerant.

Today some areas that are largely lactose intolerant are South America, Africa, and China. Over 90% of the Chinese are lactose intolerant. By contrast, only 4% of Sweden's population is lactose intolerant. In America, lactose intolerance varies by race with 14% of Caucasians being intolerant, and 74% of African Americans having difficulty with lactose.

One thing that distinguishes humans is that we can eat almost anything. That allows us to thrive anywhere we go. However, once we settle in a place, our genes change to adapt to that food source.

Where did your ancestors come from? Consider trying that diet. Was it rich in plants? Did your ancestors eat dairy? How much meat do you think they ate?

One thing we know for sure, we did not develop eating the current Western diet of burgers, fries, and pizza. That diet is killing people all over the world who are abandoning their indigenous diets and now are eating sugar, wheat, and processed oils.

Interesting milk facts: About 80% of the protein in milk is called casein. The other 20% is the more familiar whey protein, the kind found in protein powders. There are two kinds of casein in milk, called A-1 beta-casein and A-2 beta-casein. Many people have digestive problems with the A-1 milk. The A-2 protein seems to be easier to digest. If you have problems digesting milk, try the A-2 variety. Raw means no homogenization or pasteurization. Raw milk is just like it comes out of the cow. Dairies that sell raw milk should advertise what kind of cow it comes from. Breeds of cows that produce A2 beta-casein are Guernsey, Jersey, Charolais and Limousin. [183]

In addition to digestive problems, A-1 casein has been linked to type 1 diabetes, heart disease, sudden infant death syndrome (SIDS), and autism. [176] This doesn't mean that it causes these diseases. The research is primarily observational, meaning that it shows correlation, not causation. More research needs to be done. However, it is something to consider when choosing milk.

What should kids eat?

Children on low-fat diets suffer from growth problems, failure to thrive and learning disabilities.
--Dr. Natasha Campbell-McBride [44]

Poor nutrition in childhood leads to the risk of high blood pressure in adulthood.
--Dr. Joseph Mercola [55]

The healthiest food for babies is breast milk. It is good for moms to nurse until the baby is at least 1 year old. Around the world it is common for babies to nurse up to age two and beyond.

Baby food is a western invention.

Children, when they are old enough for food, should be eating the same healthy foods that their parents eat. Many people think that their children will not eat healthy foods. However, consider that children from Japan eat seaweed and raw fish. Children from Korea eat foods that are so hot that most Americans couldn't eat it. Kids will eat what they are given to eat, and they will want to eat what their parents are eating.

What do children need for health and normal growth?

They need a good balance of

- Healthy protein (meat, eggs, and fish)
- Healthy carbohydrates (fruits and vegetables)
- Healthy fat (avocados, eggs, fatty meats, grass-fed cheese, whole milk– unless they do not tolerate milk well)
- Enough vitamins and minerals in these foods

What should they avoid?

- Sugar (spikes blood sugar and very little nutrition)
- Flour (spikes blood sugar and very little nutrition)
- Deep-fried foods (unhealthy oils – trans fats)
- Most vegetable oils (olive oil and coconut oil are OK)
- All packaged and processed foods if they are made with the above ingredients

Giving them a good variety of healthy foods is the key to having healthy children. **They don't have any different needs for types of foods than adults do.**

How much should they eat?

Babies and toddlers will let you know when they are hungry and when they have had enough food. Every child has a sense of his or her own hunger. Let them eat the amount they want, and when they want it. If they don't feel like eating, or are only eating a small amount, let them decide. Babies and toddlers should be offered food at least every 3 hours.

However, only let them choose from healthy foods.

Do your best to:

- Keep family meals pleasant and positive.
- It is best if you set a good example for eating a variety of healthy foods. They want to do what you are doing.
- Make physical activity part of your family life. Going to the park,

taking walks, throwing balls, tag, etc. can be fun family activities.
- Make sure they get enough sleep. Make bedtime a pleasant experience, so they go to sleep feeling relaxed and loved. Have bedtime routines, and try to make bedtime approximately the same time each night. Exceptions are fine occasionally.

Should you avoid feeding them sugar altogether?

Babies are born liking things that are sweet. However, it is important that they eat a variety of nutritious foods. They will often choose sweet foods if they can eat whatever they want.

Until a few hundred years ago, eating too much sugar wouldn't have even been an issue. Sugar was not available in abundance. Even fruit was only available a few months a year.

However, now eating sugar is an issue.

Some parents choose to feed their children no sugar at all. That is very healthy for the children, but perhaps hard to continue once they start school and come into contact with other children who are eating an abundance of sugar and flour.

I think the best thing is to have lots of healthy choices available for children.

It is best if the parents can be a good example for healthy eating. I know this is hard, but they are watching and copying.

What is the problem with children eating poorly?

They may experience some of these things:

- Growth and development may suffer.
- They may have less energy.
- Academic and athletic performance may suffer.
- They may become anxious or depressed.
- They may have trouble focusing (brain fog).
- They may have trouble relaxing (being agitated).
- They may be underweight or overweight.
- Their immune systems may suffer, so they may have more illnesses.
- They may have trouble sleeping.
- They may have digestive problems, such as diarrhea, constipation,

244

irritable bowel syndrome, and acid reflux.
- They may have an increased risk for heart disease, high blood pressure, or type 2 diabetes later in life. [24]
- They may develop autism or hyperactive disorders.

What are the typical problems with getting children to eat healthy food?

- They want the same limited range of foods every day.
- Sometimes they refuse to eat entire food groups, such as vegetables or meat.
- Eating foods with very little nutrition

What should we avoid feeding our children, and why

- Sweetened oatmeal (oatmeal is OK, but not the sugar)
- Sweetened yogurt (yogurt is OK, but not the sugar)
- Mac and cheese (very little nutrition)
- Candy (sugar)
- Sweet rolls (sugar and flour)
- Doughnuts (sugar, flour, and deep-fried)
- Cookies (sugar and flour)
- Crackers (flour, spikes blood sugar)
- Fake cheese (very little nutrition, and artificial ingredients)
- Deep fried chicken pieces (anything deep-fried is bad)
- French fries (deep-fried, very little nutrition, potatoes spike blood sugar)
- Burgers (it is the bun that is the biggest problem here, spikes blood sugar, and ketchup has too much sugar)
- Pizza (very little nutrition, flour spikes blood sugar, processed meats, like pepperoni, are unhealthy)
- Non-fat milk (they need the fat)
- Cereal (sugar, flour, and artificial ingredients)
- Pancakes (sugar, flour, and very little nutrition)
- Pasta made from flour (spikes blood sugar, very little nutrition)

Many of these are thought of as "kid foods" but they are exactly what **kids should not be eating.**
It is possible to make healthy substitutions to these popular

foods. For example:

- **Oatmeal can be eaten with nuts, seeds, raisins, fresh fruit, and whole milk. Hot or cold. No sugar.**
- **Burgers can be eaten without the bun, with grass-fed beef, organic tomatoes and avocado, and grass-fed sour cream, lettuce and spices. Or burgers can be made using "bread" without flour, using only healthy ingredients.**
- **Gouda cheese from grass-fed cows for healthy fat and vitamin K2 (helps make healthy teeth and bones) is a cheese kids might like.**
- **Pasta can be made from quinoa (really a seed).**
- **Pancakes can be made from 1 banana and 2 eggs in a blender with blended fruit for syrup (or no syrup at all).**

What should they be eating?

A variety of fruits and vegetables. All colors. Preferably organic. Preferably seasonal and locally grown. Try everything. Ask them to eat one bite. It often takes many "tastes" before a child accepts a new food.

If you are not used to eating this way, you may want to try it, too. Tastes do change as you get used to a new food. **Even "picky eaters" will adjust if you only give them healthy alternatives.**

If that seems too difficult, at least limit their sugar intake. Sugar is the food that is making us so sick, and causing most modern diseases. Eliminating added sugar for only 9 days profoundly improved obese children's illnesses. [29]

I know this may be easy to say, but hard to do.

However, if children are hungry enough, they will eat healthy food.

Just like adults, their gut bacteria adjust over a very short period of time. Our gut bacteria may have a huge impact on what we want to eat. If you can get them through the first week, and are consistent after that, the children should just go along with the program.

There are situations that make this system harder. One of them is divorce. If one spouse wants the children to eat healthy food, and the other feeds the children sugar, flour, and junk food, that is a problem. In this case, the children become addicted to the sugar and flour, so their little bodies are craving these all the time.

However, in families where the parents can control what the children eat, do your best to feed them healthy food. Even if the parents are dealing with their own food issues, they can still feed the children in a healthy way.

I heard a story about a little girl who went to school for the first time. Her parents only fed her healthy food. She came home and told her parents that all of the other kids ate sandwiches with white bread, and ate potato chips and cookies. Then she said to her parents, "Don't those parents love their children?" That's not what I expected her to say. Good for her!

Do not feel guilty if you have not been feeding your children an ideal diet. The American culture supports feeding children sugar and processed foods. These unhealthy foods are everywhere. You might try making changes gradually if an abrupt change seems too jarring.

Sugar

"Children who eat a high amount of sugar have an increased likelihood of becoming obese adults. That puts them at risk of developing type 2 diabetes, heart disease and certain cancers . . .

"When children eat an abundance of sugar, the damage to the metabolism is brutal and happens early. If it's not corrected before age 2, we can't correct it later. That is why good nutrition is so important at an early age."

Vivien Altman [24]

Let's hope that second part is not true (if it is not corrected before age 2). I believe that it is never too late to start on a healthy diet.

Do children need cholesterol?

- The developing brain and eyes of the fetus and newborn infant require large amounts of cholesterol. Breast milk has a large percentage of cholesterol. [185]
- Children deprived of cholesterol in infancy may end up with poor eyesight and brain function. [44] [52]
- Sadly, most infant formulas follow the anti-cholesterol dogma and provide almost no cholesterol in their products. [138]

Does healthy food cost too much?

Maybe you think it costs too much to feed an entire family with healthy food. **Food is not the place to economize.** Economize on housing, cable TV, or cars, but not on food.

Keep in mind that in 1900, before modern farming equipment, about 50% of the population were farmers. Now it is less than 2%. Food, compared to 1900, is incredibly cheap.

Maybe you are comparing the dollar meals at the local fast-food burger place with healthy food. However, if you add up what you really spend on food, you might be surprised at how much you spend. For many households, buying healthy foods and cooking at home is actually cheaper than buying the pizzas, burgers and fries that many families are eating now.

In addition, you need to add:

- The cost of medical bills when you and your family get sick
- The cost of medicine
- Lost wages for time out when sick
- Lower productivity because you and your family members don't feel alert and energetic.
- The damage to the environment that conventional foods create, such as pesticides in our food and water.
- And, worst of all, the long-term damage to the bodies of your little children who may not be getting adequate nutrition to develop properly.

Bottom line, the place to economize is not on food.

(Personal Note)

When I was growing up, my mother didn't allow us to have bread in the house. Also, no potato chips, no cookies, no candy, no ice cream, no cake, no sweet rolls, etc. What did we do for lunch at school? We took "birdie sandwiches". These were a lettuce leaf with meat, cheese, tomato, a pickle, mayonnaise and mustard, with a tooth pick through it to keep it together. We added an apple, banana or an

orange, and that was lunch. I think my siblings hated this, but I liked it. Like it or not, we all did it. We ate meat, vegetables, fruit, and dairy. That's about it. No sugar or flour. No potatoes. (OK, there were some exceptions.)

It can be done, but parents have to think it is important.

Take Away

- We each inherited specific genetic programming from our ancestors. This includes what foods we can digest well. Where were you ancestors from? What did they eat? Try eating that.
- Babies and children should be eating the same healthy foods that adults should be eating. All packaged and processed foods should be limited or eliminated.
- Sugar, flour, and vegetable oils are just as unhealthy for kids as they are for adults.
- Kids and adults do best on real organic foods.
- Food is not the place to economize.
- Even picky eaters can learn to enjoy healthy foods, even vegetables. Their bodies will lose their cravings for sugar and flour after they are eliminated from their diets.
- Getting enough healthy cholesterol is important for babies and kids.

Chapter 11

What Else Besides Food

Exercise

We've all heard that "exercise is good for you", but do you know exactly why? Many people may say that it is important for weight loss. **It actually isn't all that effective for losing weight.** Walking up 8 flights of stairs only burns about 20 calories. Certainly, you burn more calories than just sitting, but changing your eating habits is much more effective for weight loss. **So why exercise?**

It keeps our bodies working. We need healthy muscles to hold our bodies together. Think about your joints. **The muscles around your joints keep them strong.** Without those muscles, the joints start to have aches and pains. You have heard of "keeping your core strong"? These are the muscles around our stomach and back. Stand up and move. Walking, lifting, virtually everything you do attaches to your core. Without a strong core, you can't make your body do what it needs to do. You start to have problems with your spine. Your posture may change. The stomach muscles keep your internal organs in the right place.

Bones also lose density with age, and lack of weight-bearing exercise plays a role in osteoporosis. Your body responds to the demands you put on it, and if you do not exercise, your muscles and bones weaken with time.

What else does exercise do?

- Exercise strengthens your **immune system**. You will get sick less often.
- Exercise can **boost your memory** and help you learn better.
- Exercise can reduce **stress.**
- Exercise can improve **sleep.**
- Exercise can boost **energy.**
- Exercise can improve **sex.** Exercise improves circulation, which is important when it comes to sex.
- You may **live longer.**
- It can make you **happier.**
- **It can reduce blood pressure** primarily by making your heart stronger.
- **It can lower type 2 diabetes risk.** By engaging in regular physical exercise, you improve your body's ability to metabolize glucose.
- It can **reduce body fat.**
- **It builds muscle mass.** With more muscle mass, your body burns more calories. Also, with more muscle mass, your body can do what you want it to do.
- **It can improve your breathing.**
- **It improves mood.** Exercise is more effective in reducing depression than medication or therapy.
- **It lowers anxiety.**
- **It can feel like fun.** Do something you love. Dancing, swimming, tennis, walking with a friend. Find something you will want to do.
- **It can reduce absenteeism.**
- **It lowers dementia risk,** primarily because you're improving the flow of blood throughout your body, including your brain.

WOW! What a list! What's not to love about exercising?!

What kind of exercise should you do?

Try to do something every day. Aim for at least one-half hour per day. At least twice a week (preferably 3 times per week), do **resistance training** (weights). That helps keep muscles strong. If you are new to exercise, try walking. If you are already fairly fit, I recommend interval training (getting your heart rate up a few times during your workout, also known as **cardio**). This doesn't have to be something difficult. Sometimes I jump (as if I am jumping rope). I jump 50-100 times. I do this 2-3 times in a workout. That gets my heart rate going! We did this for fun as kids. Pretend you are having fun. **Stretching** is the other thing to do to complete your workout. This keeps your joints in good working order.

Question: There is one exercise that is far superior to all of the others. Do you know what it its?

Answer: It's the one you will do. Find out what that is for you. Maybe that is dancing, swimming, or a competitive sport (my personal favorites). Maybe it is walking with a friend, or through the shopping mall. Maybe you like exercise classes.

Here is a list of possible exercises.

Pick one that looks like fun to you:

- Tennis
- Racquetball
- Pickleball (popular with seniors)
- Dancing
- Swimming or water aerobics
- Running (can be tough on the joints)
- Walking -- at the mall, at the beach, around your neighborhood or through a large store if the weather is bad
- Golf, especially without a cart
- Hiking -- as you age, pick trails with good footing
- Frisbee
- Basketball
- Volleyball
- Jumping rope, or just jumping
- Walking the dog -- everything counts
- Work out at the gym -- machines, classes, swimming, cycling, or hire a personal trainer
- Yoga -- can be great for stretching and resistance, but usually not so good for cardio
- Badminton

It is best to do a range of things that include all three types of exercise: stretching, cardio (heart beating faster) and resistance (weight training).

Check out my YouTube videos on exercise.

Sleep

Get at least 7 hours of sleep a night.

Sleep is just as important as the food you eat, maybe even more important. It is essential that we go through a complete sleep cycle. It is during the REM (Rapid Eye Movement) phase of sleep that recovery of our mind and body occurs. If people don't get adequate REM sleep, they have mental and physical ailments.

What happens if we don't get enough sleep?

Our "circadian rhythm" is "our 24-hour internal clock that cycles between sleepiness and alertness at regular intervals. It's also known as your sleep/wake cycle." [186]

Our need for sleep changes as we age. As newborns, we need 14-17 hours of sleep, teens need 8-10 hours of sleep, adults need 7-9 hours, and seniors need 7-8 hours.

Every bodily function is impacted if we don't get enough sleep.

Suggestions to improve sleep

- Light is a major factor in regulating sleep. It is best to have a very dark bedroom. You may need to add blackout curtains and eliminate all electronics that add light.
- Exercising in the morning outside in the sun is a great way to start your day. Morning exercisers sleep better than people who exercise later in the day. Exercising 30 minutes daily improves sleep.
- Drink liquids early in the day, and limit liquids in the evening, so that you do not have to get up to use the bathroom at night. However, if you are sleeping deeply, your body is supposed to slow down urine production, so you can sleep through the night.

- Stop eating at least 3 hours before going to bed. Raising blood sugar interferes with sleep. In addition, digesting food during sleep interferes with our body's ability to do its work of healing our cells.
- Our bedroom should be reserved for sleeping (and sex). Avoid eating, working, or watching TV in the bedroom.
- Before electricity, we went to bed soon after sunset and woke up at sunrise. Our bodies are set for this cycle. We seem to get our best sleep between 10 pm and 2 am, or some say between 11pm and 1am. In any case, set a sleep schedule and stick to it. This makes it easier for your body to fall asleep and wake up. It is best to keep the same schedule even on weekends.
- Have a bedtime ritual. I like to do stretches before I go to bed. Find something that relaxes you.
- Move all electronics at least 3 feet away from your bed to reduce EMF exposure (just in case).
- Do not deal with anything negative right before bedtime. Instead, have some bedtime ritual that is pleasant and calming, and helps clear your mind of negativity. It can be as simple as listing everything you have to be grateful for every night.
- Avoid alcohol. Alcohol may help you go to sleep, but it can interfere with your sleep cycle. Many people who drink before going to bed wake up after the alcohol wears off, and then cannot go back to sleep.
- Avoid caffeine. Even an afternoon coffee drink can interfere with sleep at night.
- Lose excess weight. Being overweight can interfere with sleep.
- Avoid all drugs. Even prescriptions drugs can interfere with sleep. Even drugs for sleeping can keep us from cycling naturally through REM.
- If you have difficulty going to sleep, try taking a hot shower or bath before bedtime. Being warm helps us fall asleep.
- Keep the bedroom cool. We sleep best if the room is between 60 and 68 degrees.
- Drinking turkey broth in the evening may help (for the tryptophan).
- Try taking a vitamin D3 supplement until your vitamin D level gets up to 50-70.
- If muscle cramps, or "restless legs" are keeping you awake, try taking a magnesium supplement.

What are the changes we experience in our sleep over a lifetime?

- Babies sleep a few hours, then wake up to eat, sleep a few hours, then wake up to eat. We don't really want to "sleep like a baby".
- Toddlers usually sleep through the night, and also take an afternoon nap.
- Teenagers go to bed later, often hate going to bed, but can't get up in the morning.
- Young adults go to bed even later (midnight or later), and want to sleep in the morning.
- Adults usually go to bed earlier and get up earlier.
- Seniors often go to bed soon after the sun sets and get up early.

Although we may have different sleep patterns as we age, it is not "normal", past the toddler stage, to have trouble sleeping through the night. If you wake up at night and can't go back to sleep, do something about it. Sleeping well has a huge impact on your health and well-being.

What about naps as adults?

Do what your body is used to. Napping is fine.

(Personal Note)

I am a napper. I don't nap every day, but I often take a nap. This has been a lifetime pattern. If I take a short nap about 5PM, or at least lie down for a short time, I have the energy to go out in the evening.

Stress

A little stress is good for us. It makes us feel excited about life. A lot of stress is bad. Try to find that happy medium. Remember that most of our stress is not coming from the outside. It is coming from inside us. It is from our attitude, or what we tell ourselves about our lives. If you don't see a way to end your stress, consider seeing a therapist.

Toxins

You might be surprised at how many toxins are in your life. Think about all of the chemicals we use every day. Read this list and eliminate as many as possible. You don't know what kind of effect they are having on you until you get rid of them.

- **Body lotion.** Read labels. You probably don't know what most of the things on the label are. I suggest buying organic lotions. Or you could try using organic coconut oil. It is not ideal because it is so oily. I make my own body lotion out of organic ingredients that I understand.
- **Soaps** (clothes, dishes, shampoo, house cleaners). Try using just water to clean your house. I use laundry soap, and dishwasher soap, only if I need it. Washing with plain water usually works fine. Most things don't really need soap. They just need to be rinsed. Also, skipping the soap is better for the environment. Soap does make things smell better. That is why some people use soap. However, even the perfumes in soaps can be toxic.
- **Make-up.** Check labels.
- **Deodorant.** I suggest using organic deodorants. I make my own from organic ingredients. It's not as effective as the chemicals, but my skin is happier.
- **Water.** 50-70 percent of rain water has roundup. Try filtered water or healthy delivered water. Avoid using disposable plastic bottles. Get water with no fluoride or chlorine, but with natural minerals.
- **Fresh air.** Go out in nature and breathe the air (beach, mountains, or the park)
- **Furniture.** New furniture often has lots of chemicals. Let it air out for a few days with the windows open. New carpet can have toxic chemicals for a few years! [44]
- **Air pollution.** Be aware of the air quality that is around you. Try not to breathe bad air. If there is a smoker around you, or exhaust from a vehicle, avoid breathing that air.
- **Pesticide drift.** If you are near a field that is being sprayed with a toxic chemical, avoid breathing it. If you live near one, consider moving.
- **Toxic mold in your home or workplace.** Check for mold. The most likely place is a drip that you can't see, such as under a sink.
- **New clothes.** Wash new clothes before you wear them. They may have chemicals on them that are toxic.

- **Electro and Magnetic Fields (EMF)** exposure is a possible area of concern. The World Health Organization (WHO) suggests that we reduce our exposure, just to be on the safe side. For example, move electronics such as alarm clocks, phones, or laptops, away from your bed at night.

Mental attitude

Our joy in life is largely based on our mental attitude, and not nearly as much on our circumstances as we might think. We have control over our mental attitude. We may have less control over our circumstances.

Bad things do happen. Sometimes bad things happen that are completely outside of our control.

I have a friend whose husband, while riding a bicycle, was hit by a drunk driver. In fact, it was a hit-and-run drunk driver. Her husband did not die, but was severely brain-damaged. It would have been easy for her to be bitter and hateful. However, she has done a remarkable job of changing her mental attitude over the years since it happened. She found out who did it, knocked on his door, and forgave him. If she can recover from that, I bet you can overcome the challenges in your life.

The point of having a better mental attitude is to have peace in our lives. If you are bitter, angry, resentful, jealous or envious of others, it damages you. If you do not have joy and peace in your life, it is much more difficult to eat healthy food and take good care of your body.

But how do you go from feeling these negative emotions to peace?

Tips for improving mental attitude

- **Practice an "attitude of gratitude".** Every day think about all that you have to be grateful for. Write them down.
- Look on the bright side.
- See the best in those around you.
- **Find the humor in everything.**
- It's not what life gives you, it's what you do with it that counts (making lemonade out of lemons).
- Care about others.
- Give to others.
- **Don't complain.** If you are having a problem, talk to a friend, but

with the attitude of solving the problem, not just complaining.

- **Our image of ourselves is based on what we get reflected back to us from other people.** So, be with people who like you. Don't spend time with people who don't like you. You will feel much better about yourself if you do.
- Not everyone is good at everything. Know what you are good at and what you are not good at. Go with your strengths. **You only need to be good at enough things, not everything.**
- **Take responsibility for everything in your life.** Don't blame others. Look at your part in what happened. It creates peace within you to do this.
- Let others be fully who they are. **Don't try to change other people.** Your choice is to be with them or not be with them, not to change them. That is their business.
- Follow the serenity prayer.
- Find a group of people who like you, and you like them. This can be a church, workplace, family, friends, or neighborhood. **Find people to care about.**
- If you have wronged someone, clear it up. If someone has wronged you, clear it up. This may mean forgiving them, or just letting go of the negative feelings. Or it might mean undoing something bad that you did (give money back that you stole).
- **Don't compare yourself to others.** You can always find someone who is better at something than you are. Let them be better. Don't let it mean anything about you. Cheer them on. Concentrate at being the best YOU that you can be.

Motivation

When I was a psychologist in private practice, after the first session with a new client, I knew whether or not the client would do well. How? Motivation. That is something I could not supply. They had to walk in the door with it. I could supply how to get there, but if they did not walk in the door with motivation, we would not go anywhere.

The same is true of being healthy. If you really want to be healthy, how to get there is known. Follow what I am suggesting and you will clear up almost all, if not all, of your health issues. Of course, if you have an advanced disease, maybe my suggestions are too late to reverse the problem. But maybe not. And, of course, some diseases are outside the range of this book (but you don't know unless you try this first).

In any case, if you bring the motivation to this project, this book supplies the rest (for most things).

Obstacles to change

If we could all be healthy by just wishing it so, we probably all would be. However, there are barriers to making changes.

Which of these beliefs may be stopping you from changing?

Unhealthy food:

- It's really **easy**
- Everyone else is eating it, so it **seems normal.**
- That is **how I was raised**, so that is what people should be eating.
- I like it. There is nothing like a cream-filled, sugar-coated deep-fried doughnut covered with chocolate frosting?

These are probably all true. That is why people eat unhealthy food. What beliefs may be stopping you from eating healthy food?

Healthy food:

- It takes **more time and effort** to shop and cook.
- You **don't know how** to shop for and cook healthy food.
- You think healthy food **won't taste good.**
- It will **cost too much.**
- **You don't believe that it will matter** all that much.
- You **don't care** enough about your health.

Or

- It just **too hard to change.**
- You are **addicted** to sugar, or flour, and processed foods, and don't want to address these issues.

Let's take these one at a time and examine them.

- It takes **more time and effort** to shop and cook.

It's hard to argue with that one. It is so easy to go through a drive-thru for burgers, fries and a soda, or a pizza. What about eating healthy foods? We have to shop. We have to know what to buy. We have to have some recipe in mind. We have to cook it. Then we have to clean the kitchen after eating. It is harder. **You have to think the extra time and effort are worth it.**

- You **don't know how** to shop for and cook healthy food.

Cooking is a learnable skill. In fact, I really enjoy cooking. Check out my YouTube videos on shopping and cooking.

Or take a healthy cooking class. You could learn how to cook and perhaps meet people to support you in your new journey.

- You think healthy food **won't taste good.**

I think this one is completely off base.

You think you won't like it, but I predict you will like it better once you and your body get used to it.

It goes like this: You start eating healthy food. Your body feels good for the first time, well, ever! You didn't realize the lethargy, aches and pains, and actual diseases were because of your food and lifestyle. After you get used to eating healthy food, when you see a piece of cake, your stomach might feel queasy. You find that you really don't want it.

You might try a dessert occasionally, just to see how it feels to eat your favorite sweets. You have a piece of cake. You feel awful afterwards, sometimes for days. You really had no idea that cake was doing this to you. Eventually, you will lose all interest in eating like that. You look forward to your delicious healthy food. You really will enjoy eating it, and come to love how good you feel afterwards.

In addition, after you cut out sugar and flour, your tastes change. Everything tastes so much better without sugar and flour – eventually.

Also, almost everything unhealthy can be made in a healthy way by substituting healthy ingredients. OK, not cake, cookies and ice cream, but there are other desserts you might find to be more delicious and satisfying. Check out my recipes.

- It will **cost too much.**

One hundred years ago, Americans spent up to 70% of their income on food. In 1915, 31% of the American workers were farmers. Today, less than 2% of workers are farmers, and food is cheaper than ever. We now spend about 10% of our earnings on food.

And yet, we complain about the cost of food. We want to eat the cheapest food available, even if it offers very little nutrition, and is full of ingredients that are slowly killing us.

Fresh organic produce, especially compared to 100 years ago, is incredibly cheap. **The place to economize is not on food.** Economize on housing, cars, TVs, entertainment, or expensive coffee drinks, but not on food.

In addition, **fast food is really not that cheap.** I bet that, for most people, buying healthy food and cooking at home may even be cheaper than eating fast food. People compare a fast-food dollar burger to healthy food, but that is not typically what people eat. It is expensive to feed a family of four at a restaurant, even a fast-food restaurant.

- **You don't believe that eating healthy won't really change your life much -- or the lives of your children.**

I hope that the information in this book will change your mind.

- You **don't care** enough about your health.

In order to make a big change, you have to want to live, want to see your kids and grandkids grow up, and want to continue to have fun with life. If life isn't valuable enough to you, take a serious look at this. See a therapist. Talk to your friends. Go to a support group. Start having more fun with life.

- It just too **hard to change.**

Most people have a very difficult time changing habits. They are used to eating certain things and find it hard to give them up. No matter how delicious the new foods may be, most people have a craving for the foods they are used to eating.

Maybe start a little at a time, gradually adding a few more healthy foods. Give your tastes a chance to adjust to the new foods.

- You are **addicted** to sugar, or flour, and processed foods, and don't want to address these issues.

You may have a sugar or carbohydrate addiction without realizing it. Making the decision to eliminate these foods, and sticking to it, may help eliminate the cravings. There are support groups if doing it alone seems too hard. You could also go to a therapist who specializes in this.

Mostly, what it takes to eat a healthy diet is to have the commitment to do it. If you are committed, the rest isn't so hard. There are solutions to every barrier. You have to believe it is worth it.

Keep in mind:

If eating unhealthy food kills your body, then where are you going to live?
--Natasha Campbell-McBride [44]

After you have made the commitment to eating a healthier diet, you may have trouble sticking to it. Try reading these every day:

Never confuse a single defeat with a final defeat.
--F. Scott Fitzgerald

It does not matter how slowly you go as long as you do not stop.
--Confucius

Fall down seven times; get up eight.
-- Japanese Proverb

I am a slow walker, but I never walk back.
--Abraham Lincoln

The man who moves a mountain begins by carrying away small stones.
--Confucius

Have a joyful life

Happy people live longer -- about 35% longer!!

Tips for having a joyful life

Track your activities for one week. After each activity, rate it 1 to 10. After a week, look at your activities. Are they mostly 3's or 8's?

As much as possible, get rid of anything under a 4. Keep everything over a 7. Do you need any of these activities that are under a 7? Sometimes you do need these. Paying bills or doing laundry may not be a very high number, but they need to be done.

Sometimes just changing your attitude can change the number. Maybe you have a low number on a certain activity. If you need to keep the activity, think about how you could change your attitude about that activity.

For example, if you think your job is boring, think about how you might see your job in a different light. You might focus on being grateful that you have a job. It pays the bills. Maybe it is good that it is boring, because that might be better than having a stressful job.

Or you might think about what you might do to make it more interesting. Maybe you could make a friend at work. Often people look forward to work because of the people, not so much the job itself.

Or you could make the work into a game. I read about a photographer who used to make the photo editing into a game. He would track how many pictures he could do in an hour. Then he would try to beat his record.

Think about how you might make your activities more fun.

Or you could change the activity to make it more enjoyable. Maybe you could listen to music while doing the laundry, or put your favorite TV show on. **I like to put the TV on while cooking. It makes cooking very relaxing and enjoyable.**

I had a friend who used to start every day by reading the news. He would get angry and depressed. One possibility is that he stop reading the news. I don't follow the daily news. I call it "the daily disaster report". All of the terrible things that happen all over the world are reported. Do we really need to know about every car accident? Take a good look at all of your activities and think about the impact they have on you.

Sometimes people just get into the **habit of having a bad time.** People seem to love to complain. This is not helpful. If you are complaining in order to solve a problem, that is fine, but if you are complaining just to complain, that is not good for you or the listener. Ideally, you would structure your life so there is really nothing to complain about. You would have lots of joyful activities, and the necessary ones that aren't so wonderful, you would have altered enough that they are not worthy of complaining.

Focus on all of the activities that are 8's, 9's, and 10's. Do more of those. Think about what other activities might be fun. Do those and rate them. Keep any that create joy.

Sometimes our circumstances are very difficult, such as the death of a child, or an illness, or an injury. This is different. We all have circumstances which are upsetting or depressing. I am not talking about that. Those things we just need to get through the best way we can. I am talking about the everydayness of life and making that better.

The people who live long, healthy lives are those who enjoy their lives. This is largely under your control. Make your life into a joyful one.

Tips for staying healthy

- Track what you eat -- try using Cronometer.com, a free website.
- Eat only organic fruits and vegetables.
- Eat organic or grass-fed animal products.
- Eat wild Alaskan Sockeye Salmon once or twice a week (3-6 oz.).
- Eat a colorful variety of fruits and vegetables.
- Eat something every day with K2.
- Get vitamin D from sunshine (not on face and hands) or from a supplement if you don't live in a sunny area.
- Get at least 7 hours of non-medicated sleep.

Love and relationships

What creates the most happiness and joy? Making money? Living in a big house? Going on exotic vacations?

Those are fine as short-term boosts, but **the real joy in life comes from our relationships.** How many good relationships do we need? I think we need just one really good one, but most people would like to have more than one person to be attached to. What would this really good relationship look like?

- You understand and accept each other.
- Perfection is not required, but acceptance of the other person is essential.
- Supporting the other person emotionally
- Be on his or her side
- Holding the other person as more important than anything or anyone else.
- As you go through life with another person, you get to see how that person behaves in different situations. Will they support you and be concerned about your joys, upsets and stresses? Will they abandon you when you need them? Will you be there for them?

But what if your special person wants you to give up every other important person in your life? Or they want you to do things that hurt your life? Not a good idea. That is when we go from being a good partner to a destructive relationship. So, don't blindly support the other person. **You have needs, too**. You have other important people in your life. However, make sure your special person feels heard, seen, and appreciated. Talk it over until you are both happy.

Relationships are what fuel everything else.

Action item:

I suggest that you make a list of what matters the most. For most people the top of the list is a person, probably a spouse, or perhaps children. However, for some people, it is work. For others it may be a hobby. I suggest that many of your problems in relationships come from this list.

If your spouse is at the top of the list, every decision throughout the day should reflect this. If your boss asks you to work late on your spouse's birthday, your answer should be clear if you want to have a good relationship with your spouse.

Even if you have a job that has irregular hours (heart surgeon, real estate agent, or police detective), your priorities need to be addressed so that your spouse does not feel neglected.

For some people an addiction, such as food, alcohol, or drugs, is at the top of the list.

Be clear about what your list is. Is it a list that supports good relationships? Is it a list that supports you having the life of your dreams?

How are we doing as a culture here in America?

I think we are not doing so well.

Why are so many people lonely?

In spite of the fact that most people live in close proximity to many other people, we don't really know each other very well.

How many true friends do you have? Who can you tell anything to and know that you will be accepted?

I have noticed that Americans are losing their ability to have nurturing conversations. Many people are "conversational narcissists". These are people who are always talking about themselves and have very little interest in what anyone else has to say.

We all want someone to listen and care, but we have to be willing to listen and care about other people, too. It has to go both ways.

When you are in a conversation, notice if you are really listening to the other person, or are you just thinking about what you will say next. If you find you are doing too much of the talking, try asking questions. Say things like, "tell me more about that", or "that must have felt awful" or "wow!" Just make a comment to let the other person know you are interested. However, **you need to actually care about what they are saying.**

If you find yourself talking to a conversational narcissist, try saying things like, "Let me finish my point."

Even if people are not good at conversation, most of us want to connect. We want to have friends who care about us. No one wants to have other people avoid us.

We can't change other people.

Old joke:

Q: How many psychologists does it take to change a light bulb?
A: Only one, but the light bulb has to want to be changed.

The same is true of our friends and family. We can't change them. Our job is to see them clearly, and love and accept them as they are.

If we really don't like someone in our lives, we can choose to not spend time with them. That's it.

There are exceptions. We can say we are worried about our loved ones. We can give them real feedback about how their behavior affects us, but we do not have the power to change other people.

Does more money make us happier?

If you do not have enough money to provide a basic living (food and shelter), then money does matter. Beyond that, money provides incrementally more happiness, but not much. If wealth provided happiness, wealthy people would not drink, do drugs, or kill themselves, but of course, they do.

Optimism helps us live longer

Having a positive outlook on life has been shown to be THE most influential factor in longevity studies. [187]

Researchers at the University College London in the United Kingdom [188] studied 9,365 adults over 50 with an average age of 63. They asked them to rate four questions on a 4-point scale. They did the ratings three times at 2-year intervals between 2002 and 2006, with a follow-up in 2013.

Sadly, they found that 24% of participants reported no high levels of life enjoyment on any occasion, and death rates in this group were the highest at follow-up.

However, 34% had ratings of high enjoyment. They had the lowest rate of mortality. In fact, it was 24% lower!

Other factors that correlated with high enjoyment of life were:

- Being female
- Married or cohabiting
- Currently employed
- Well-educated
- Wealthier
- Younger. [116]

Being optimistic reduces illnesses.

Author Julia Boehm, from the Harvard School of Public Health, found "that factors such as optimism, life satisfaction, and happiness are associated with reduced risk of CHD regardless of such factors as a person's age, socioeconomic status, smoking status, or body weight."

In addition, Dr. Linda Sowpresa found that positive thinking impacted longevity of humans more than any other factor.

In the Nurses' Health Study, a study tracking women's health over many years, it was found that the most optimistic women had a nearly 30 percent lower risk of dying from any cause compared to the least optimistic.

More specifically, the most optimistic women had a:

- 16 % lower risk of dying from cancer.
- 38% lower risk of dying from heart disease.
- 39% lower risk of dying from a stroke.
- 38% lower risk of dying from respiratory disease.
- 52% lower risk of dying from infection.

The good news is that being optimistic is largely under our control. We can decide to see things from a positive viewpoint. We make this choice just as we make the choice to eat healthy food or to exercise regularly. Choosing to adopt an optimistic attitude can change your life profoundly. **Positive emotions are generated by the thoughts we think. We have control over those thoughts.**

Thinking positive thoughts not only helps us live longer, but positive thoughts generate positive emotions. Having control over being able to generate positive emotions is one of the greatest gifts you can give yourself. Changing our thoughts can be a simple as seeing the best way a situation can turn out rather than dwelling on how many things can go wrong.

Gratitude

If I had to give only one suggestion to improve health and happiness, it would be to have an **attitude of gratitude**. Every day, be grateful for what you have. Make a list and say it out loud. For example:

I am grateful that I am healthy.
I am grateful to be alive.
I am grateful for my home.
I am grateful for the food I eat.
I am grateful for the people in my life.
I am grateful for the activities I have.
I am grateful for the opportunities in my life.
I am grateful for the sunshine or the weather.

Every day, add the specifics for that day. Make the list real for yourself. Keep making the list until you truly feel the gratitude.

If you find yourself feeling resentful, angry, jealous, or any other negative emotion, let it go as best you can. Focus on the positives in your life.

Everyone is given some positive traits, and some negative traits. Focus on the gifts you have. Don't focus on the things you don't have. Don't compare yourself to others.

I think that luck is random, good and bad luck. However, we have a huge amount of control over our environment by the energy and attitude we put out into the universe. The happy, friendly person generally has a much easier time negotiating through life than the grumpy negative person. We like to interact with happy, cheerful people. We like to help happy, cheerful people. Try being that person.

I know this sounds trite, but the truth is that lives well-lived focus on being the best YOU that you can be.

Take Away

- **Food is the major contributor to good health. However, there are other important factors to consider. These are sleep, stress, toxins, and mental attitude.**
- **Relationships are our most powerful motivating force. If these are going well, it is much easier for us to take good care of ourselves. Create good relationships around you.**
- **I think the easiest and most powerful change you can make to improve your health is to have an attitude of gratitude (OK, that and taking vitamin D and eliminating sugar). Stop complaining. Focus on what is good in your life. Just being alive is a gift!**

Chapter 12

My Favorite Recipes

"The food you eat can be either the safest and most powerful form of medicine or the slowest form of poison."
--Dr. Ann Wigmore

"Learn how to cook –try new recipes, learn from your mistakes, be fearless, and above all, have fun!"
--Julia Child

These are some of my favorite recipes. Check out my other book, **Easy Keto Recipes**, *Lose Weight Without Hunger*. After doing the research for this book, I developed an eating system that reflects what I learned. I have included almost everything I eat in my recipe book. In addition, I have included a picture for almost every recipe.

Everything you eat should be in the service of keeping you healthy. Most people don't think of food this way. They eat whatever is convenient, or cheap, or what they feel like eating. Instead, **consider what your body needs to stay healthy and make sure that you get enough of these things every day. In addition, eliminate everything that hurts your body.** With this in mind, here are some recipes to get you started.

Use organic ingredients whenever possible.

Only ten recipes

Dr. William P. Castelli, director of the Framingham Heart Study, after evaluating 5,000 people for almost 30 years, said that **most people rotate through only 10 recipes throughout their lives.**

If we really only eat 10 recipes throughout our lives, then changing our eating habits should be fairly easy. **Just find 10 healthy recipes that you really love, and eat them.** [169]

These are the recipes that I use. I don't eat anything that I don't love. I show how to make these on my cooking videos on YouTube under *Andrea Covert* **or** *Creating Health.*

Cooking essentials

To enjoy cooking, these are 3 essentials.

- **Sharp knives.** I have one serrated knife (useful when a "grip" is required, as with onions) and one rocker knife (perfect for cutting vegetables into smaller pieces), both very sharp.
- **A large cutting board.** I use a large wooden cutting board. It's easy on the sharp knives. Plastic and bamboo are too hard. If you oil the wooden cutting board regularly, it will last a very long time.
- **A good pan.** I use good quality ceramic pans. The food doesn't stick and it washes with a soft brush. I have been using the same one for years, and it is still like new. The ceramic should not scratch or come off in your food. If it does, buy a better pan. Don't wash it with soap. Don't put it in the dishwasher. It needs a good coat of oil to keep it working well. After all, you are going to be cooking with it, so you don't need to worry about bacteria. Do not use Teflon, which can be carcinogenic. Do not us aluminum. This is a poison that can come off in your food. Stainless steel is great as long as you are not frying. It tends to stick. A good brand for ceramic pans is Green Pan, available on Amazon.

Check out my YouTube videos to see me making these recipes.

Meat

All animals should be raised outdoors, eating what they are meant to eat. They should not be fed GMO corn or soy grown with pesticides or herbicides. Also, no growth hormones or antibiotics.

That said, pick the meat you like.

The easiest way to fix any meat is as follows:

I take out the amount I am going to eat. I slice the meat into 1/2 to 1 inch pieces. I put the sliced meat in a pan with a small amount of coconut oil or animal fat, and spices. My favorites are bacon fat (organic) and Kinder's prime rib seasoning.

Cook chicken and pork just until they are no longer pink in the middle. If you overcook these, they will be dry and tough. Cook beef until it is how you like it (as in pink for medium-rare). This only takes a minute or two. It is a very fast meal!

If the meat produces excess liquid, pour this off. I put it on my plate and use it as a sauce. If the liquid stays in the pan, the meat won't brown.

That's it. Eat it by itself, or add it to soups, salads, or vegetables. My favorite meat: steak cooked in a pan with bacon pieces and fresh garlic.

Greek Fritata -- Quiche Without a Crust

A delicious way to eat a variety of vegetables
1 large onion, chopped
1 large tomato, chopped
1 tbsp. coconut oil or bacon fat
2 cups of spinach, uncooked and chopped
8 eggs from pastured-fed chickens
2 cups shredded Gouda cheese from grass-fed cows
½ cup pitted Greek olives (optional)
1 tsp. Dash's Lemon Pepper
1 tsp. Italian seasoning mix
2 cups of your favorite vegetables, cut up and cooked, such as broccoli,

carrots, leeks, fennel, Brussel sprouts, or mushrooms.
1 cup total of your favorite fresh herbs, such as cilantro, dill, or basil. Use 1
tbsp. of dried if you don't have fresh. This is optional.

Preheat oven to 375 degrees.

Put onions and tomatoes into pan with coconut oil with half of the spices. Add the other vegetables. Do not overcook. Add spinach and fresh herbs. Cook just long enough to wilt them. Put all of the vegetables into small glass casserole dishes, or one large casserole dish. Add olives and cheese to dishes.

Put eggs into a bowl and mix. Add the rest of the spices. Pour over vegetables in the casserole dish.

Bake for 30- 45 minutes or until frittata is firm and lightly brown on top.

Bone Broth

I eat this every week to keep my joints healthy.

What bones to use:

Use bones from animals raised on organic healthy food. Do not use bones from animals that have been on the feed lots and have been fed GMO corn and soy, or with added hormones and antibiotics.

Use 3 pounds of any combination of these: chicken backs, chicken necks, chicken feet, chicken wings, and any chicken bones you have saved up in the freezer. Turkey necks and backs work well, too. Beef, pork, or lamb bones can also be used. Pig's feet are good. Sometimes I buy a whole chicken (organic), cut off the legs and breast meat, and use the rest for bone broth.

Put these in the water with the bones:
8 cloves of organic garlic
2 tbsp. of lemon juice

I like these spices, but use the ones that are your favorites, or whatever you have. Don't add too much. You can always add more later.

10 cups of healthy water, (no chlorine or fluoride), enough to cover the ingredients

You can use a slow cooker or a pressure cooker, or cook on the stove. I like to put the ingredients into my Instant Pot cooker and cook on "slow cook" for 24-48 hours. If you cook it on the stove, it should be cooked on low (barely boiling) for 12-24 hours.

After cooking, put it through a strainer to get rid of all of the solid food. Throw this away. However, if you are recovering from digestive disorders, keep the meat and vegetables and eat them with the broth. They are very easy to digest. They have very little nutrition at this point, and are rather tasteless, but easy on the digestive system.

You can drink it just like this, or use it for a base in soups or other dishes.

Chicken and pork feet: Why? Bone broth is a great source of collagen, and the feet are an especially rich source of collagen. Collagen makes your joints healthier, helps reduce wrinkles, increases the gut lining (so it helps with things like leaky gut, IBS, Crohn's disease, ulcerative colitis and acid reflux), boosts metabolism, and strengthens teeth and nails. I think bone broth is a major factor in keeping my joints pain-free.

This same recipe can be used for any other bones (beef, lamb, etc.), but you should cook them longer (perhaps 48 hours), because the bones are tougher.

I save broccoli stems, fennel tops, asparagus tough ends, cauliflower leaves and tough bottoms, and any other "throw away" parts of veggies I buy, put them in the freezer, and cook these in my bone broth. They are still delicious and full of nutrition, even if they are too tough to eat. I usually have so many of these that I do not need to add any more veggies. In addition, it has so much flavor this way that I just add sea salt. No other spices. Done this way, made with "throw -away" veggies and bones, it is practically free.

Green Beans

I pound of green beans
1 tbsp. coconut oil or bacon fat
¼ tsp. Dash's lemon pepper
1/4 tsp. Kinder's lemon pepper
2 cubes of frozen lemon juice, or juice of 2 lemons

Cut off the stem end of the green beans. I like to cut the beans up into 1-2-inch sections, but this is not necessary.

Put all ingredients in a frying pan. Cook on medium heat.

Cook until beans are tender. This may be only 10 minutes, but some green beans are tough and need up to 30 minutes of cooking. In addition, sometimes green beans have a sharp bitter taste. Usually cooking more gets rid of this flavor.

I make a huge amount and refrigerate whatever I don't eat. I usually eat a mix of vegetables every day and green beans are a great addition to that mix.

One way to encourage kids to eat veggies is to tell them to eat these like French fries, and dip them the sour cream (1 cup) and barbecue sauce (1 tbsp.). You might need to start with more barbecue sauce in the beginning.

Haas Avocado

I love these. I either eat them plain, or add Himalayan sea salt, or a spice such as Kinder's lemon pepper, or a bit of flavored Balsamic vinegar.

They have very healthy oil. We need oil, but it should be healthy oil. Avocados are also a great source of magnesium, a very important nutrient, especially for older people who may have trouble metabolizing it. I typically eat 1/3 avocado every day. They are also great in salads, or as a topping on salmon or eggs.

When I buy avocados, I leave some out to ripen, and put the rest in the refrigerator. They take about 2 days to ripen at room temperature, so as I eat them, I take a few more out of the refrigerator.

Avocados turn brown when exposed to the air, so if I don't eat the whole avocado, I put it in a cup, cut side down, so the air cannot get to it. That way, it is still fresh the next day.

Desserts

Yogurt and Fruit

1/2 cup full-fat Grass-fed Greek yogurt
½ cup blueberries, blackberries, strawberries, or a mix
Add a sprinkling of nuts and seeds on top.
Add cinnnamon
1/2 tsp honey (optional)

Put in a dessert cup. Yum!

Chocolate Fat Bombs

These are high in fat, but low in carbs. I eat these for the magnesium, and as a healthy treat after a meal. The molds I use are 1 tsp, which has only 1 gram of carbohydrates. Pretty good for a yummy end to a meal.

1/2 cup organic coconut oil, melted
1/2 cup grass-fed butter, melted (1 cube)
1/2 tsp vanilla
1 cup organic cacao powder (my favorite is Navitas)
1/4 cup raw honey
1/8 tsp Himalayan salt
1 1/2 cups of organic nuts and seeds. Choose your favorites.
Seeds: Chia seeds (adds a crunchiness, and for the omega 3's), hemp seeds (tastes like walnuts but without the bitterness), pumpkin seeds, cashews (chopped), almonds (chopped), pecans (chopped). These are easily chopped in a coffee grinder or food processor. I buy all of the nuts at Costco.
Note: I make a large batch of chopped nuts, store them in the freezer, and use them over time in different foods.

Melt the butter and coconut oil in a pan. Add the honey, salt, and vanilla. Put hot ingredients in a mixing bowl. Add cacao powder and nuts. Taste it. The only unhealthy ingredient in this is the honey (because it is sugar), so use as little as possible. Use just enough to make it taste good to you. Honey is a real food, but it is still sugar.

Put these in soft silicon molds and store them in your refrigerator.

Chocolate is very healthy. It has lots of magnesium. Chocolate is generally thought to be unhealthy because of the ingredients that are usually added to chocolate, such as sugar.

Coconut oil is very healthy. One part of coconut oil is called MCT (Medium Chain Triglyceride) oil, which is very good for our brains, especially in preventing Alzheimer's.

Almonds are considered the healthiest nut. They are packed full nutrition such as magnesium, vitamin E and healthy fat. They help reduce hunger. However, most nuts and seeds are good for us, so use your favorites.

When I am losing weight, and keeping my net carbs under 10, I eat these yummy chocolate fat bombs after meals to reduce hunger. It works for me. I think it is best to limit these to 5-10 teaspoons per day. One gram of carbohydrate per teaspoon.

(Personal Note)

What does a typical day of eating look like for me?

I often start my day by eating one third of an avocado (for the fats and magnesium). I eat this with 1 tbsp. of Gouda Cheese, (for the K2) and perhaps some fresh microgreens, (full of micronutrients). This is my first food of the day, usually about 11 am.

About 2 PM, I eat my main meal, which is a large mix of vegetables with meat or eggs. Sometimes just veggies. Sometimes mainly meat. I eat just until I am full. This should last until the next morning, but in case I am hungry at night, I have a small amount to eat. I might have some nuts, or a bowl of soup. I don't eat within 3 hours of sleeping.

I typically drink bone broth, water, mineral water, or herb tea for hydration. I aim for 40-60 oz. of water, often with LMNT added for minerals. It has magnesium, potassium, and salt.

This system of eating has kept me extremely healthy over the years. I am now 75. I am 5"6", and usually weigh 115-120 pounds. I take no medication. I have no aches or pains. I have abundant energy, and I choose to believe that my brain still works well.

I wish you the best on your journey to health and longevity!

You might want to look at my YouTube videos about:

- **What I do to exercise (swimming and pool exercises, stretching and yoga)**
- **How to cook delicious healthy food**
- **Talks about health and nutrition**
- **Conversations with kids and adults about eating healthy food**

You can find these on YouTube: Creating Health with Dr. Andrea Covert

My other book,

Easy Keto Recipes: Lose Weight Without Hunger,

Has pictues for almost every recipe.
I developed these recipes to go along with this book to
make it easy to put these principles into practice.

Appendix A

15 Things to boost your immune system

These are things you can do to avoid getting sick, or only have a mild case of any illness.

Read the list. Do the things you are willing to do. Everything helps.

People die of diseases, not necessarily because of the disease itself, but because the individual does not have a healthy immune system to fight the disease. Which changes would you be willing to do? Try doing that.

If you want to do one really easy thing, take vitamin D until your vitamin D level gets to 50-70 ng/ml. Ask your doctor to do a blood test to see what it is now. People with higher vitamin D levels were far less likely to get sick or die of Covid. I took 10,000 IU for several months, until my level reached 70 ng/ml, then I took less (3,000 IU per day).

I am not a physician and am not giving medical advice. This is just information for you to consider.

1. Eat real foods

Real foods are those that nature made, not processed or in a package. Recommended foods are:

- Non-starchy organic vegetables, in a range of colors.
- Whole fruits, no fruit juice.
- Limit very sweet fruits, such as grapes and pineapple.
- Limit starchy vegetables like potatoes.

2. No sugar or artificial sweeteners.

- I know this seems very difficult, but try it.
- Your tastes will adjust.

3. Eat enough protein.

Eat about one third to half of your body weight in grams (40-60 grams for a 120-pound woman). That is a piece of meat about the size of the palm of your hand. Recommended proteins are:

- Grass-fed meats, 3-6 oz per day, with fat
- Fish low in mercury, such as wild-caught Alaskan Sockeye salmon, 3-6 oz. per week
- Nuts and seeds
- Non-GMO soy
- Eggs from pasture-fed hens. For example, 1 egg is 6 grams of protein.

4. Eat healthy fats

Do not eat any bean and seed oils, such as canola oil, soybean oil, Crisco, or safflower oil. Healthy fats are:

- Avocados
- Nuts and seeds, which are also a good source of magnesium
- Eggs from pasture-fed hens
- Animal fats from grass-fed animals
- Olive oil
- Coconut oil
- Cheese from grass-fed cows, which is also good for Vitamin K2

5. Add super-healthy foods

Garlic, onion, berries, mushrooms, and spices are packed with nutrition. Add these to soups, vegetable dishes, and sauces. Sprouts of all kinds, such as broccoli, kale, mustard, and radish, have far more nutrition than the adult vegetable.

6. Eat Fermented foods.

- These add to your gut microbiome.
- Your gut microbiome is a major part of your immune system. Fermented foods help increase the diversity of your healthy gut bacteria.
- Eat foods that are naturally fermented. My favorite is sauerkraut, but not the kind in a can. Look for naturally fermented foods.

They should be in the refrigerated section.

- Unsweetened yogurt (full-fat and pasture-fed) and kefir are also good.

7. Make bone broth from grass-fed animals.

- Bone broth gives a big boost to your immune system. It is also good for your joints.

8. Hydrate, especially with water.

- My favorites are herb tea, or water with a cube of lemon juice.
- Avoid fruit juices and all sweetened beverages.
- Avoid all sodas, even with artificial sweetener.
- Drink water without fluoride or chlorine and with natural minerals.

9. Avoid grains, alcohol, and processed foods

- Grains and all grain products, including flour, bread and pasta (I know this seems difficult and extreme, but it can make a huge difference, just like eliminating sugar)
- Alcohol
- All processed foods (packaged foods)

10. Give your digestion a break

- When you eat may be just as important as what you eat.
- Finish eating in the afternoon, then don't eat again for at least 12 hours, preferably 16 hours. This gives your digestion a rest, and allows your body to do its "housekeeping". A 16-hour break could be from 6 PM to 10 AM, for example.

11. Get enough sleep.

- Get 7-9 hours of sleep per night, without sleep medication.
- Sleep may be even more important than nutrition.
- Establish a bedtime ritual.
- Go to bed at the same time each night.
- Do something relaxing before bed, such as stretching or

meditation
- This is a good time to review everything you are grateful for.

12. Exercise daily, 30-45 minutes.

- Do something every day
- Don't overdo it because that stresses the immune system.

13. Take supplements

- Vitamin D

More than 80% of the US population has insufficient vitamin D. [189] Vitamin D is instrumental in many of our body's processes. As people age, our bodies don't process vitamin D as well, so we may need to take a supplement.

"Studies have shown that people with vitamin D deficiency are 11 times more likely to get a cold or flu, while supplementing with vitamin D can reduce colds and flu by 42%." [189]

Foods high in vitamin D are wild-caught salmon, herring, sardines, egg yolks, and mushrooms.

- Magnesium

About 75% of the US population is deficient in magnesium. Like Vitamin D, magnesium is instrumental in many of our enzymatic reactions. Taking magnesium, or soaking in Epson salts before bed, helps our muscles relax. Foods high in magnesium are spinach, pumpkin and chia seeds, cacao, bananas and avocados.

If you get leg cramps, that is a sign that you may need more magnesium.

- Vitamin C

Helps the immune system stay strong.

However, the best source of vitamin C is food. For vitamin C to work well, it needs a complex of nutrients that come together in a package in real food. Supplementing with vitamin C is fine for a short-term boost, but for the long-term, eat real food. Foods high in vitamin C are: yellow and red bell peppers, kiwi, broccoli, Brussel sprouts, strawberries, oranges, cauliflower, and cabbage. [190]

14. Wash your hands

- Bacteria and viruses get into our bodies primarily through our mouth, nose and eyes.
- Wash your hands after coming into contact with possible disease-causing agents
- Don't touch your face.

15. Stop Smoking

- This would be a great time to stop
- The coronavirus attacks the lungs.

By contrast, what do Americans typically eat?
63% is processed (packaged) food which is primarily flour, sugar, and unhealthy oils (bean and seed oils). These have calories but very little nutrition, and are toxic to our bodies.

Appendix B

Printable summary

What to Eat on a Ketogenic Diet

Do not eat these foods

- Processed and packaged foods
- Processed carbohydrates, such as cereals, bread, pasta, and rice
- Processed meats – such as salami, hot dogs, bacon, sausages, and luncheon meats (some of these can be healthy if made from grass-fed animals and are cured without adding toxic chemicals)
- Any form of sugar, such as table sugar, honey, any form of syrup, sucrose, fructose, dextrose, maltose, or rice sugar.
- Flour from any grain, even whole grain flour
- Soda, any kind, with sugar or artificial sweeteners
- Trans fats
- Deep-fried foods
- Most vegetable oils - corn, soybean, canola, cottonseed, sunflower, safflower, sesame, grapeseed, rapeseed, and rice bran oil, or anything with "partially hydrogenated"
- Read the ingredients on everything. If you don't know what an ingredient is, or can't pronounce it, don't buy the product. The ingredient is probably an unhealthy chemical.

Eat these – Preferably organic

- Non-starchy vegetables – unlimited amounts – a variety of colors – raw and cooked- should be about 80% by volume of what you eat
- Fruit, especially berries – large range but limited quantity due to the sugar content
- Wild Alaskan Sockeye Salmon - 1-2 times per week – 3-6 oz per serving
- Grass-fed full-fat dairy (cheese - Gouda is best, sour cream,

cream cheese, yogurt) – limited amounts due to high calorie count – some every day for vitamin K2.

- Nuts and seeds – every day - good variety but not too much due to high calorie count
- Garlic
- Turmeric
- Dark chocolate, small amounts – daily up to 1 square OK, 70% cacao or more (less sugar)
- Cook with coconut oil or add to dishes – aim for 1-2 tablespoons per day
- Extra virgin olive oil in limited amounts due to high calorie count. Do not cook with this.

Controversial foods:

- Milk has lactose (sugar), and many people have problems digesting it, so limit or eliminate this if there are problems.
- Grass-fed or pasture-fed meat only, but how much? From none to lots
- Beans, limited amounts or none at all
- White potatoes, occasionally or not at all
- Sweet potatoes. Healthier than white potatoes, but high in carbs, so limited amount

Other essential non-food items:

- Drink water – with minerals but no chlorine or fluoride
- Get adequate sunshine every day for Vitamin D (or take a supplement)

Why eat these?

- **Non-starchy vegetables**

You can eat these in unlimited amounts
Eat a variety of colors – raw and cooked
Good source of micronutrients and fiber
Easy to feel full because of unlimited volume

Should be 80% in volume of daily food

- **Fruit, especially berries**

Eat a large range but limited amounts due to high sugar content
Good source of micronutrients and fiber
Adds delicious taste to dishes, or good for dessert
Eat primarily low-sugar fruit

- **Wild Alaskan Sockeye Salmon**

Eat this 1-2 times per week, 6 oz per serving
Good source of omega 3 fatty acids; excellent source of protein, B vitamins, including B12, and minerals, especially selenium and phosphorus. Has lots of Vitamin D.

- **Grass-fed full-fat dairy**

This includes cheese (Gouda is best), sour cream, cream cheese, yogurt, and eggs
Limited amounts due to high calorie count
Some every day for vitamin K2 and vitamin B12;
Excellent source of complete protein, B vitamins, folate, vitamins A and C
Fats help us feel full

- **Nuts and seeds**

Eat some every day. Eat a good variety but not too much due to the high calorie count.
Good source of omega 3, protein, copper, iron, magnesium, manganese, phosphorus, and zinc.
Studies show that people who eat nuts and seeds daily live up to 7 years longer.

- **Garlic**

Garlic has many medicinal qualities. It boosts the immune system, improves blood pressure and cholesterol levels, has antioxidants that may prevent Alzheimer's disease and dementia.

It is packed with nutrition, such as manganese, calcium, copper, potassium, phosphorus, iron and vitamins B1 and B6, vitamin C, selenium, and fiber.

It is delicious in soups, sauces, dressings, and many other foods.

It is most effective when cut up or crushed right before eating with minimal cooking.

Eat fresh garlic for best results. Cut up and let sit for 10 minutes before cooking.

Eat raw mint, apples, or lettuce with garlic to minimize garlic breath.

- **Turmeric (Curcumin)**

This is an extremely effective nutritional food.

It helps prevent heart disease, Alzheimer's and cancer.

It's an anti-inflammatory and antioxidant.

It improves depression and arthritis.

Works best when eaten with pepper.

- **Sweet potatoes**

This has anti-inflammatory and anti-oxidant properties.

In spite of being a starchy root vegetable, they help stabilize blood sugar.

It has lots of vitamin A (beta-carotene), potassium, vitamin C, fiber, niacin, vitamins B1, B2, B3, B6, phosphorous, manganese, copper, pantothenic acid, and biotin.

- **Dark chocolate**

Eat this in small amounts, such as one square daily, that is 70% cacao or more.

Excellent source of antioxidants, like flavonoids.

Chocolate helps with cardiovascular health, has diabetes protection, anti-cancer benefits, and is good for bone health, and brain health.

Contains fiber, iron, magnesium, copper, manganese, potassium, phosphorus, zinc, and selenium.

However, it is highly acidic (cancer likes this)

It can dehydrate.

Contains caffeine which may be connected to breast cancer.

- **Coconut oil**

Cook with this or add it to dishes. Aim for 1-2 tablespoons per day.
MCT oils (Medium Chain Triglycerides) are instrumental in reversing or preventing Alzheimer's. Coconut oil is part MCT oil.
Coconut oil has a very high burn temperature, so it is safe to use in cooking (does not oxidize or turn into trans fats at high temperatures).

- **Extra virgin olive oil**

Eat this in limited amounts due to high calorie count.
Do not cook with this.
Some researchers believe that olive oil is a key ingredient in the success of the Mediterranean Diet.
It gets rancid fairly quickly, so eat within a few months of purchase, and make sure that it is fresh when you buy it.

- **Grass-fed meat and fat**

Eat only grass-fed and grass-finished organic meat.
Eat only pasture-fed chickens and eggs.
These are a good source of protein and vitamin B12.
Healthy fats are good for you.

- **White potatoes**

Eat these occasionally or not at all.
Starchy vegetables are filling and delicious.
However, they have limited nutrition and spike blood sugar.
They have a higher Glycemic Index than sugar.
They are OK occasionally, especially when eaten with other things that reduce the glycemic load.
Not recommended if you are on a high-fat diet

- **Drink water**

Drink water with minerals but with no chlorine or fluoride.
Fluoride and chlorine are poisons. They should be filtered out of

your water. However, if you filter everything out, you are left with no minerals.

Minerals found in spring water are very healthy for us.

We are about 60% water, and it is essential for every cell of our bodies to have adequate water.

There is no agreement about how much water should be consumed daily (the most common suggestion is 64 oz. per day). However, this may not be science-based.

Eating organic fruits and vegetables containing water is an excellent source of hydration

Dental health has a huge impact on general health.

- Use a soft toothbrush and change it frequently.
- Floss daily.
- Use a chemical-free toothpaste (no fluoride).
- Get regular dental checkups.

Action Item

Get unhealthy food out of your kitchen.

If you want to be healthy, take all unhealthy food out of your kitchen. What foods to eliminate:

- All wheat products, such as bread, pasta, tortillas, pretzels, crackers, and packages of macaroni and cheese
- All breakfast cereals that have any sugar or flour (probably all of them)
- All condiments that contain sugar, artificial ingredients, or unhealthy oil. That includes ketchup, mayonnaise, barbecue sauce, soy sauce, and most mustards. Costco now sells some healthy organic condiments that are fairly low in sugar.
- All fruit juices, because of the sugar content.
- Rice (spikes blood sugar)
- Instant oatmeal (because of the sugar and artificial ingredients)
- Jams, jellies, and pancake syrup
- All cooking oils that are unhealthy, especially corn oil, safflower

oil, canola oil, sunflower oil, and soybean oil. Olive oil, avocado oil, and coconut oil are fine.

- Packaged frozen dinners, including frozen pizzas
- Processed meats (hot dogs, sausage, spam, lunch meats, etc.) unless they are made from grass-fed animals, have no added unhealthy ingredients such as nitrates and nitrites, and are uncured
- Packages of potato chips, and tortilla chips
- Anything with sugar, such as cookies, cakes, ice cream, and candy
- Any sweetened drinks
- Anything with artificial sweeteners, including drinks
- Artificial cheeses, such as American Cheese and Velveeta
- Most canned foods (some few are OK – read the label)

You can sometimes have these in your kitchen, but don't eat them very much or very often:

- Potatoes
- Organic corn, fresh or frozen
- Alcohol (research is mixed)

If you are really serious about your health, also eliminate all forms of sugar, including:

- Honey (this is the only "real food")
- Maple syrup
- Agave

For those of us who love our desserts, I know that this last one is pretty extreme. It is hard to think about giving up all forms of sugar. But the thought is actually harder than doing it. If you eliminate all sugars and sweeteners for two weeks, you will probably lose, or at least minimize, your cravings for sweets. Try it. It's only two weeks. Take it one day at a time. At the end of each day, ask yourself how hard that was. Do one more day. Each day gets easier until you lose your cravings for sweets. I love my desserts. This worked for me. Now I love eating desserts without sugar. Check out the dessert section of this book.

Bibliography

[1]	D. Buettner, The Blue Zones Solution, Washington, D.C.: National Geographic Society, 2015.
[2]	C. M. Benbrook, "Trends in glyphosate herbicide use in the United States and globally," 02 February 2016. [Online]. Available: https://enveurope.springeropen.com/articles/10.1186/s12302-016-0070-0.
[3]	J. Fung, The Obesity Code Cookbook, Vancouver/Berkeley: Greystone Books, 2019.
[4]	N. McCarthy, "The Top New Year's Resolutions For 2019," 2 January 2019. [Online]. Available: https://www.statista.com/chart/16500/top-us-new-years-resolutions/. [Accessed 04 May 2021].
[5]	J. Fung, The Obesity Code Unlocking the Secrets of Weight Loss, Canada: Greystone Books, 2016.
[6]	A. e. a. Stunkard, "An adoptive study of human obesity," Vols. Jan 26: 314 (4):193-8, 1986.
[7]	A. e. a. Stunkard, "The body-mass index of twins who have been reared apart," *New England J of Med.*, pp. May 24: 322(21):1483-7., 1990.
[8]	N. White, "Influence of intensive diabetes treatment on body weight and composition of adults with type 1 Diabetes Control and Complications Trial," *Diabetes Care,* pp. 24(10):1711-21, 2001.
[9]	L. e. a. Kong, "Insulin resistance and inflammation predict kinetic body weight changes in response to dietary weight loss and maintenance in overweight and obese subjects by using a Bayesian network approach," *Am. J Clin Nutr,* pp. 98(6):1385-94, 2013.
[10]	F. e. a. Cappuccio , "Meta-analysis of short sleep duration and obesity in children and adults," *Sleep,* pp. May;31(5):619-26, 2008.
[11]	C. A. Knobbe, "Diseases of Civilization: Are Seed Oil Excesses the Unifying Mechanism?," in *Low Carb Denver 2020*, Denver, Colorado, 2020.
[12]	D. Ludwig, Always Hungry?, New York, New York: Grand Central Life and Style, 2016.
[13]	J. DiNicolantonio, The Salt Fix Why the Experts Got It All Wrong -- and How Eating More MIght Save Your LIfe, New York: Harmony Books, 2017.
[14]	D. J. Mercola, Fat for Fuel: A revolutinalry Diet to Combat Cancer, Boost Brain Power, and Increase Your Energy, Carlsbad, California: Hay House, Inc., 2017.
[15]	A. Blazyte, "Average per capita sugar consumption in urban households in China from 2013 to 2018," 25 November 2019. [Online].
[16]	J. Fung and J. Moore, The Complete Guide to Fasting Heal Your Body Through Intermittent, Alternate-Day and Extended Fasting, Canada: Victory Belt Publishing, 2016.
[17]	J. Mercola and B. Bikman, "Physiological Effects of the Ketogenic Diet With Dr. Benjamin Bikman," [Online]. Available: https://youtu.be/YRfaHC75Cr0.
[18]	J. Mercola, Ketofast Rejuvinate Your Health with a Step-by-step Guide to Timing Your Ketogenic Meals, Carlsbad, CA: Hay House, 2019.
[19]	K. Loria, "The True Story of a Man Who Survived Without Any Food For 382 Days," 2 March 2017. [Online]. Available: https://www.sciencealert.com/the-true-story-of-a-man-who-survived-without-any-food-for-382-days.
[20]	Stewart, W.K. and L. W. Fleming, "Features of a successful therapeutic fast of 382 days' duration," *Postgraduate Medican Journal,* pp. 49, 203-209, 1973.
[21]	M. Hyman, Food what the Heck should I eat?, New York: Little, Brown and Cmpany, 2018.
[22]	CDC, "Adult Obesity Prevalence Maps," 29 October 2019. [Online]. Available: https://www.cdc.gov/obesity/data/prevalence-maps.html.
[23]	J. Fung, The Cancer Code A Revolutionary New Understanding of a Medical Mystery, New York,NY: HarperCollins Publishers, 2020.

[24]	V. Altman, Director, *Globesity: Fat's New Frontier.* [Film]. 2012.
[25]	D. Daszkowski, "How American Fast Food Franchises Expanded Abroad," 11 November 2018. [Online]. Available: thebalancesmb.com.
[26]	A. Blazyte, "Average per capita sugar consumption in urban households in China from 2013 to 2018," 25 November 2019. [Online]. Available: statista.com/statistics.
[27]	10 Oct. 2017. [Online]. Available: http://dx.doi.org/10.1016/SO140-6736(14)60460-8.
[28]	6 Apr 2016. [Online]. Available: http://dx.doi.ort/10.1016/SO140-6736)16)00618-8.
[29]	R. Lustig, "Robert Lustig - What is Metabolic Syndorme Anyway?," 1 February 2019. [Online].
[30]	J. M. Esselstyn, Prevent and Reverse Heart Disease, 2007.
[31]	K. Rheaume-Bleue, Vitamin K2 and the Calcium Paradox How A Little-Known Vitamin Cound Save Your Life, Toronto, Ontario, Canada: Collins, 2012.
[32]	K. Linares, "What is Lard, and Is It Healthy? Here is What a Registered Deititian Says," 23 July 2020. [Online]. Available: https://www.prevention.com/food-nutrition/a33407032/what-is-lard/.
[33]	P. J. S. M. F. S. Bowden, The Great Cholesterol Myth Why Lowering Your Cholesterol Won't Prevent Heart Disease -- And The Statin-free Plan That Will, Beverly, MA: Fair Winds Press, 2012.
[34]	D. M. Herrington, et al., "Dietary Fats, Carbohydrate, and Progression of Coronary Atherosclerosis in Postmenopausal Women," *American Journal of kClinical Nutrition 80,* pp. No. 5 1175-84, 2004.
[35]	F. B. Hu et al., "Meta-analysis of Prospective Cohort Studies Evaluating the Association of Saturated Fat with Cardiovascular Disease," *American Journal of Clinical Nutrition 91,* pp. No 3: 502-9, 2010.
[36]	R. e. a. Kuipers, "Saturated Fat, Carbohydrates, and Cardiovascular Disease," *Netherlands Journal of Medicine ,* pp. 69, no. 9: 372-78, 2011.
[37]	G. Taubes, Why We Get Fat and What To Do About It, New York, New York: Alfred A Knoff, 2011.
[38]	V. Stefansson, Not by Bread Alone, New York: repr., Macmillan, 1956, 1946.
[39]	N. Teicholz, The Big Fat Surprise Why Butter, Meat & Cheese Belong in a Healthy Diet, New York, NY: Simon & Schuster, 2014.
[40]	J. Bowden, Living the Low Carb Life From Atkins to The Zone, New York: Sterling Publishing Co., Inc., 2004.
[41]	G. V. Mann, R. D. Shaffer and R. S. Anderson, "Cardiovascular Disease in the Massai," *Journal of Atherosclerosis Research,* pp. 289-312, 1964.
[42]	A. Hrdlicka, "Physiological and Medical Observations Among the Indians of Southwestern United States and Northern Mexico," U.S. Government Printing Office, Washington, D.C., 1908.
[43]	Mayo Clinic Staff, "Peritonitis," [Online]. Available: https://www.mayoclinic.org/diseases-conditions/peritonitis/symptoms-causes/syc-20376247.
[44]	N. Campbell-McBride, Put Your Heart in Your Mouth, United Kingdom: Medinform Publishing, 2007.
[45]	T. J. Key, P. N. Appleby, E. A. Spencer, R. C. Travis, A. W. Roddam and N. E. Allen, "Mortality in British Vegetarian: Results form the European Prospecrive Investigation tinot Cans=cer and Nutrition," *American Journal of Clinical Nutrition,* pp. 89, No. 5: 1613S-1619S, 2009.
[46]	M. Hyman, Eat Fat, Get Thin Why the Fat We Eat Is the Key to Sustained Weight Loss and Vibrant Health, New York, NY: Little, Brown and Company, 2016.
[47]	L. Keith, The Vegetarian Myth food justice, and sustainability, Oakland, CA: PM Press, 2009.

[48]	B. Sanders, "Despite what you'be been told COWS CAN SAVE THE WORLD," 17 October 2020. [Online]. Available: https://www.youtube.com/watch?v=VYTjwPcNEcw&feature=youtu.be. [Accessed 15 Jan 2021].
[49]	S. e. a. Hudley, "Health polcy on blood cholesterol. Time to change directions.," *Curculation*, pp. 1026-1029, 1992.
[50]	D. Graveline, Lipitor -- thief of memory, statin drugs and the misguided war on cholesterol., Haverford, Pennsylvania: Infinity Publishing, 2006.
[51]	J. S. O'Brian and M. T. Murray, "Lipid composition of the normal human brain: gray mater, white matter and myelin," *Journal of Lipid Research*, p. Vol. 6, 1965.
[52]	K. Moore and T. Persaud, The Developing Human -- Clinical oriented embryology. 9th edition., USA: Saunders, an imprint of Elservier Inc., 2011.
[53]	U. Ravnskov, The Cholesterol Myths. Exposing the fallacy that saturated fat and cholesterol cause heart disease., New Trends Publishing, 2000.
[54]	C. e. a. Iribarren, "Cohort study of serum total cholesterol and in-hospital incidence of infectious disesases.," *Epidemiology and Infection*, pp. 121, 335-347, 1998.
[55]	J. Mercola, 20 April 2016. [Online]. Available: https://articles.mercola.com/sites/articles/archive/2016/04/20/cholesterol-myths.aspx. [Accessed 6 May 2021].
[56]	V. Marigliano and et al., "Normal values in extreme old age," *Annals of eh New York Aademy of Scineces 673*, pp. 23-28, 1992.
[57]	H. M. E. S. Taylor FC, "Statin therapy for primary preventin of cardiovascular disease.," *JAMA*, pp. 310 (22) 2451-52, 2013.
[58]	J. Simmons, "The $10 billion Pill," *Fortune*, pp. 147 (1): 58-62, 66, 68, January 2003.
[59]	D. Lundell, "The Truth About Heart Disease & Cholesterol," [Online]. Available: https://youtu.be/8A-BEm8xtW0.
[60]	J. Mercola, "Fructose: The Hidden and Pervasive Cause of High Blood Pressure," 22 July 2010. [Online]. Available: https://articles.mercola.com/sites/articles/archive/2010/07/22/high-fructose-diet-contributes-to-high-blood-pressure.aspx.
[61]	D. Graveline, "spacedoc.net," 2008. [Online].
[62]	P. Y. Lee, K. P. Alexander, B. G. Hammell, S. K. Pasquali and E. D. Peterson, "Representation of Elderly Persons and Women in Published Randomized Trials of Acutr Coronary Symdormes," *Journal of the American Medical Association*, pp. 286, No. 6, 708-713, 2001.
[63]	C. M. Flavell, "Women and Coronary Heart Disease," *Progress in Cardiovascular Nursing*, pp. 9, No. 4. 18-27, 1994, Fall.
[64]	W. B. Kannel, "Metabolic Risk Factors, for Coronary Heart Disease in Women: Perspective from the Framingham Study," *American Heart Journal 114, no. 2*, pp. August, 413-419, 1987.
[65]	T. Gordon, W. P. Castelli, M. C. Hjortland, W. B. Kannel and T. R. Dawbet, "High Density Lipoprotein as a Protictive Factor Against Coronary Heart Disease: The Framingham Study," *American Journal of Medicine*, pp. 62, no 5 :707, 1977.
[66]	R. H. Knopp, B. Retzlaff, C. Walden, B. Fish, B. Buck and B. McCann, "One-year Effects of Increasingly Fat-Restricted, Carbohydrate-Enriched Diets on Lipoprotein Levels in Free-Living Subjects," in *Proceedings for the Society of Experimentl Biology and Medicine*, 2000.
[67]	D. Feldman, "Dave Feldman - It's about Energy, Not Cholesterol," 20 Jan 2018. [Online]. Available: youtube.com/watch?v=kDOHwOqhTOA$feature-youtu.be.
[68]	D. Feldman, "Dave Feldman - "New Data on Energy, Exercise, and Cholesterol"," 17 Aug 2019. [Online]. Available: youtube.com/watch?v=kDOHwoqhTOA&feature=youtu.be.
[69]	G. Taubes, Why We Get Fat and What to do About It, New Youk and Canada: Random House, 2011.
[70]	E. Woolley, "Starchy Vegetables land How to Enjoy Them," 11 September 2020. [Online]. Available: https://www.verywellhealth.com/list-of-starchy-vegetables-1087454. [Accessed 13 October 2020].

[71]	USDA, "Dietary Guidelines for Americans," Unitee States government, December 2015. [On-line]. Available: -guidelines/resources-everyone/tools-individuals-and-families. [Accessed 20 November 2020].
[72]	R. Esselstyn, The Engine 2 diet: The Texas Firefighter's 28-day Save-Your-Life Plan that Lowers Cholesterol and Burns Away the Pounds, Grand Central Life and Style, 2017.
[73]	R. Heidrich, A Race for Life, NY, NY: Lantern Books, 2000.
[74]	A. Ziehl, D. D. Thilmany and W. J. Umberger, "A Cluster Analllyses of Natural Beef Product Consumers by Shopping Behavior, Importance of Production Attributes, and Demographics," *Journal of Food Distribution Research, 36, 1,* pp. 209-217, 2005.
[75]	K. Gunnars, "11 Proven Health Benefits of Chia Seeds," 8 August 2018. [Online]. Available: https://www.healthline.com/nutrition/11-proven-health-benefits-of-chia-seeds. [Accessed 10 April 2021].
[76]	G. Taubes, The Case Against Sugar, Canada: Alfred A Knopf and Afred A Knopf, 2016.
[77]	J. Fung, The Diabetes Code Prevent and Reverse Type 2 Diabetes Naturally, Canada: Greystone Books, Ltd., 2018.
[78]	J. Yudkin, Pure, White, and Deadly How Sugar Is Killing Us and What We Can Do to Stop It, New York, New York: Penguin Group, 1972.
[79]	R. MacKarness, Eat Fat and Grow Slim, 1958.
[80]	Harvard Medical School, "Glycenic index for 60Plus foods," 14 March 2018. [Online]. Available: Health.harvard.edu.
[81]	Weight Loss for All, "Weight Loss for all.com," [Online]. Available: weightlossforall.com.
[82]	"The University of Sydney," 26 November 2019. [Online]. Available: glycemic index.com.
[83]	D. E. Bredesen, The End of Alzheimer's The First Program to Prevent and Reverse Cognitive Decline, New York, New York: Penguin Ramdom House LLC, 2017.
[84]	P. Shewry, "Wheat," *J Exp Botany,* pp. 60 (6) 1537-53, 2009.
[85]	W. Davis, Wheat Belly, New York, New York: Rodale, 2011.
[86]	B. Harper, The Skinny Rules, New York: Random House, 2012.
[87]	P. R. Mason, "Are you smarter than a Doctor?," 2019. [Online]. Available: lowcarbdownunder. com.au.
[88]	Z. e. a. Harcombe, "Evidence from Randomised Controlled Trials Did Not Support the Introduc-tion of Dietary Fat Guidelines in 1977 and 1983: A Systematic Review and Meta-analysis," *Open Heart,* pp. 2, no. 1 DOI: 10.1136/openhrt-2014-000196, 2015.
[89]	Center for Disease Control and Prevention, Division of Diabetes Translatoin, "Long-term Treads in Diabetes," 2016. [Online]. Available: https://www.cdc.gov/diabetes/statestics/slildes/long_term_trends.pdf.
[90]	F. Lipman, 10 Reasons Y/carlsbad, ou Feel Old and Get Fat . . . and How You Can Stay Young, Slim, and Happy, Carlsbad, California: Hay House, Inc., 2015.
[91]	F. Mather, "Waste Products: Cottonseed oil," *Popular Science Monthly,* p. 104, May 1894.
[92]	S. Gokhale, "Marketing Crisco," 25 June 2013. [Online]. Available: https://www.westonaprice. org/health-topics/modern-foods/marketing-crisco/.
[93]	E. McCollum, The Newer Knowledge of Nutrition: The Use of Food for the Preservation of Vital-ity and Health, Macmillan via INternet Archive, 1918.
[94]	S. Gerrior and L. Bente, "Nutrition Content of the U.S. Food Supply, 1909-1999: A summary Report.," Washington, DC: US Department of Agriculture, Center for Nutritin Policy and Promotion, 2002., Wanshinton, DC, 2002.
[95]	K. M. Anderson , W. P. Castelli and D. Levy, "Cholesterol and Mortality: 30 years Follow-up from the Framingham Study," *Journal of the American Medical Association 257, no.16 ,* pp. 2176-2180, April 24, 1987.

[96]	D. J. Fung, "Get Rid of Excess Sugar!," 25 May 2020. [Online]. Available: https://www.youtube.com/watch?v=e1R_VG9hT6w.
[97]	Cronometer, "Cronometer," 2020. [Online]. Available: Cronometer.com. [Accessed 1 May 2021].
[98]	M. Enig, "The Weston A. Price Foundation," 31 December 2001. [Online]. Available: https://www.westonaprice.org/health-topics/childrens-health/fat-and-cholesterol-in-human-milk/. [Accessed 11 March 2021].
[99]	USDA, "Dietary Guidelines for Americans, 2020-2025," 2020. [Online]. Available: https://www.dietaryguidelines.gov/sites/default/files/2021-03/Dietary_Guidelines_for_Americans-2020-2025.pdf. [Accessed 11 March 2021].
[100]	S. Ekberg, "6 Best Secrets To Reverse Insulin Resistance Naturally & Change Your Life," 31 May 2019. [Online]. Available: https://www.youtube.com/watch?v=xcQUghF2SKY. [Accessed 28 April 2021].
[101]	R. N. Proctor, "The history of the discovery of the cigarette -- lung cnacer link: evidentiary traditions, corporate denial, global toll," PubMed.gov, 21 (2): 87-91 Mar 2012. [Online]. Available: https://pubmed.ncbi.nlm.nih.gov/22345227/. [Accessed 11 March 2021].
[102]	D. Buettner, The Blue Zones, 2008.
[103]	United Nations - World Population Prospects, "U.S. Life Expectancy 1950-2020," 5 12 2020. [Online]. Available: <a href='https://www.macrotrends.net/countries/USA/united-states/life-expectancy'>U.S. Life Expectancy 1950-2020</a>. www.macrotrends.net. Retrieved 2020-12-05..
[104]	*Pittsburgh Tribune,* 2005.
[105]	P. Saladino, The Carnivore Code, United States of America: Fundimental Press, 2020.
[106]	E. R. S. USDA, 2009.
[107]	Wikipedia, "Oldest People," 7 April 2020. [Online]. Available: https://en.wikipedia.org/wiki/Oldest_people.
[108]	H. Brueck and S. Lee, "How long it takes your body to regrow 19 types of cells and organs, from your skin to your skeleton," 8 May 2018. [Online]. Available: https://www.businessinsider.com/how-long-it-takes-the-body-to-grow-hair-nails-cells-2018-4.
[109]	A. Ernst and J. Frisen, "Adult neurogenesis in humans -- common and unique traits in mammals," *Plos Biol.,* p. 13 (1):e1002045, 2015.
[110]	BiologyWise, "Parts of a Cell," [Online]. Available: https://biologywise.com/parts-of-cell.
[111]	P. Hinckey, "Autism Prevalence Increasing," 12 June 2013. [Online]. Available: https://www.behaviorismandmentalhealth.com/2013/06/12/autism-prevalence-increasing/. [Accessed 6 May 2021].
[112]	K. Thornburg, "The epidemic of chronic disease and understanding epigenetics," 28 July 2015. [Online]. Available: https://www.youtube.com/watch?v=ReCvreRPdeY.
[113]	S. e. a. Grundy, "Diagnosis and management of the metabolic syndrome: an American Heart Association/National Heart, Lung, and Blood Institute Scientific Statement.," Circulation, 2005.
[114]	G. e. a. Reaven, "Insulin resistance as a predictor of age-related diseases.," vol. 86 (8), 2001.
[115]	B. Bikman, Why We Get Sick, Dallas, Texas: BenBella Books, Inc., 2020.
[116]	M. NIchols, N. Townsend and P. Scarborough, "Cardiovascular disease in Europe: epidemological update.," *Euro Heart J.,* p. Oct., 2013.
[117]	S. Sinatra and J. C. Roberts, Reverse Heart Disease Now, Hoboken, New Jersey: John Wiley & Sons, Inc., 2007.
[118]	A. D. Sniderman, G. Thanassoulis, K. Williams and Et al, "Risk of Premature Cardiovascular Disease vs teh Number of Premature Cardiovascular Events," *JAMA Cardiol.,* pp. 1 (4): 492-494, 2016.
[119]	Guyton and Hall, Textbook of Medical Physiology, Sanders Elservier U.S. , 2011.

[120]	Doll, R. and Peto, R., "The Causes of Cancer: Qualitative Estimates of Avoidable Risks of Cancer in the United States Today",," *Journal of the National Cancer Institute 66,* pp. no. 6: 1191-1308, 1981.
[121]	T. Tsujimoto, H. Kajio and T. Sugiyama, "Assiciation between hyperinsulinemia and increased risk of cancer death in nonobese and obese peple: A population-based observational study," *Int J Cancer,* pp. 141(1): p, 102-111, 2017.
[122]	M. E. a. Bodmer, "Long-term metformin use is associated with decreased risk of breast cancer.," *Dibetes Care,* pp. 33(6): p. 1304-8, 2010.
[123]	P. e. a. Goodwin, "Fasting insulin and outcome in earlypstage breast cancer results of a prospecrie hhoort study.," *j Clin Oncol,* pp. 20(1): p. 42-51, 2002.
[124]	e. a. Sherwin R.W., "Serum cholesterol levels and cancer mortality in 361,662 men screened for the multiple risk factor intervention trial.," *Journal of the American Medical Association,* pp. 257, 943-948, 1987.
[125]	C. R. e. a. Marinac, "Prolonged Nightly Fasting and Breast Cancer Prognosis," *JAMA Oncology 2 no. 8 August 1,* pp. 1049-55 doi: 10.1001/Jamaoncol.2016.0164, 2016.
[126]	K. e. a. Katachi, "Preventive Effects of Drinking Green Tea on Cancer and Cardiovascular Disease: Epidemological Evidence for Multiple Targeting Prevention," *Biofactors,* pp. 13 nos. 104 49-54, 2000.
[127]	L. A. e. a. Mucci, "Familial Risk and Heritability of Cancer among Twins in Nordic Countries," *JAMA,* pp. 315, no. 1 68-76 January 5, 2006.
[128]	I. Raabinowitch, "Clinical and Othere Observations on Canadian Eskimos in the Western Arctic," *Canadian Medical Association Journal,* p. 34 ; 487, 1936.
[129]	O. e. a. Schafer, "The Changing Pattern of Neoplastic Disease in Canadian Eskimos," *Canadian Medical Association Journal,* pp. 112:1399-1404, 1975.
[130]	J. Friborg and M. Melbye, "Cancer Pattterns in Inuit Populations," *Lancet Oncology,* pp. 9, no.9 ;892-900, 2008.
[131]	J. Peto, "Cancer Epidemiology in the Last Century and the Next Decade," *Nature,* pp. 411, no. 6835, May 17, 390-95., 2001.
[132]	S. e. a. Basu, "The relationship of sugar to population-level diabetes prevalence: an economic analysis of repeated cross-sectional data.," vol. 8(2):e57873. doi: 10.1371/journal. pone.0057873, 2013.
[133]	P. M. Attia, "When does heart disease begin (and what that tells us about prevention)," 27 June 2016. [Online].
[134]	P. Attia and J. Fung, "Jason Fung, M.D.: Fasting as an antidote to obesity, insulin resistance, T2D, &metabolic illness," 11 January 2020. [Online]. Available: youtube.com/watch?v=nqBkGO-ZECn8.
[135]	L. Cordain, The Paleo Diet.
[136]	T. Wahls, "Minding your mitochondria	Dr. Terry Wahls	TEDxIowaCity," 30 November 2011. [Online]. Available: https://www.youtube.com/watch?v=KLjgBLwH3Wc&t=738s.
[137]	D. G. Amen, M.D., "Change Your Brain Change Your Body," Hdarmony Books, New York, 2010.
[138]	N. Campbell-McBride, Gut and Psychology Syndrome, Cambridge, UK.: Medinform Publishing, 2010.
[139]	M. Newport, Alzheimer's Disease: What if there was a cure?: The story of ketones, April 1, 2013.
[140]	D. Perlmutter, M.D. and Kristen Loberg, Grain Brain, THe Surorisig Truth About Wheat, Carbs, and Sugar -- Your Brain's Silent Killers, New York: Little, Brown and Company, 2013.
[141]	J. Mercola, "Articles.mercola.com," 22 May 2014. [Online].
[142]	S. Miyagi, N. Iwama and K. Hasegawa, "Longevity and diet in Okinawa, Japan: the past, present, and future.," *Asia Pac J Public Health,* pp. 15 Suppl: S3-9, 2003.

[143]	L. Cordain, M. hurtado and et al., "Acne vulgaris: A disease of Western civilization," *Arch Dermatol,* pp. Dec. 138:1584-90, 2002.
[144]	E. Bendiner, "Disastrous trade-off: Eskimo health for white civilization," *Hasp Pract,* pp. 156-89, 1974-9.
[145]	P. Steiner, "Necropsies on Okimawans: anatomic and pathologic observatioins," *Arch Pathol,* pp. 42:359-80, 1946.
[146]	O. Schaefr, "When the Eskimo Comes to Town," *Nutr Today,* pp. 6:8-16, 1971.
[147]	C. Adebamowo, D. Spiegelman, F. Danby and et al., "High school deitary dairy intake and teenage acne," *J Am Acad Dermatol,* pp. Feb;52 (2): 207-14, 2005.
[148]	R. Smith, N. Mann, A. Braue and et al., "A low-glycemic-load diet improves symptoms in acne vulgaris patients: a randomized controlled trial.," *Amer J clin Nutr,* pp. Jul;86(1): 107-15, 2007.
[149]	A. Jacob, Digestive Health with REAL Food: a practical guide to an anti-inflammatory, low-irritant, nutrient-dense diet for IBS & other digestive issues, Paleo Media Group LLC, 2013.
[150]	L. E. Eklund, Director, *Food As Medicine.* [Film]. 2016.
[151]	G. Fettke, "Dr. Gary Fettke -- Nutrition and Inflammation," Low Carb Down Under, 23 June 2017. [Online]. Available: https://www.youtube.com/watch?v=iCQmfRMwHfA. [Accessed 10 May 2021].
[152]	American Heart Association, Commplete Guide to Women's Heart Health, New York: Random House, 2009.
[153]	J. Mercola, Effortless Healing, United States of America: Harmony Books, 2015.
[154]	K. Rheaume-Bleue, Vitamin K2 and the Calcium Paradox.
[155]	A. Denio, "Vitamin D Deficiency: The Silent Epidemic of the Elderly," 17 December 2012. [Online]. Available: iscd.org/publications/osteroflash/vitamin-d-deficiency-the-silent-epidemic-of-the-elderly.
[156]	B. K. Harbolic, "Vitamin D Deficiency," [Online]. Available: medicinenet.com/vitamin_d_deficiency/article.htm.
[157]	M. Holick, The Vitamin D Solution.
[158]	J. Mercola, 28 May 2014. [Online]. Available: articles.mercola.com/sites/articles/archive/2014/05/28/vitamin-d-deficiency-signs-syptoms.
[159]	C. Dean, The Magnesium Miracle, Baltimore Books, 2007.
[160]	J. Garrow, Human nutrition and dieretics, 10th edition, Churchill Livingstone, 2000.
[161]	J. Mercola, "Is Magnesium the Missing Link in Your Heart Healthy Routine?," 16 January 2017. [Online]. Available: articles.vercola.com.
[162]	R. Swaminathan, "Magnesium Metabolism and its Disorders," *US National Library of Medicine National Institutes of Health,* p. May 31, 2014.
[163]	National Institute of Health, "Magnesium," 25 September 2020. [Online]. Available: https://ods.od.nih.gov/factsheets/Magnesium-HealthProfessional/#h10. [Accessed 11 February 2021].
[164]	J. Hibbeln, L. Nieminen, W. Lands, A. Tjonneland, K. Overvad and et al., "Linoleic acid, a dietary n-6 polyunsaturated fatty acid, and the aetiology of ulcerative colitis: a nested case-control study within a European prospective cohort study.," no. Dec.:58 (12):1602-11, 2009.
[165]	CDC, "Get the Facts: Sodium and the Dietary Guidelines," October 2017. [Online]. Available: https://www.cdc.gov/salt/pdfs/sodium_dietary_guidelines.pdf.
[166]	R. Bayer, D. Johns and S. Galea, "Salt and public health: contested science and the challenge of evidence-based decision making," *Health Aff (Millwood),* pp. 31 (12): 2737-2746., 2012.
[167]	N. Grausal, A. Galloe and P. Garred, "Effects fo sodium restriction on blood pressure, renin, aldosterone, catecholamines, cholesterols, and riglycerides: a meta-analysis.," Vols. 279(17): 1383-1391, 1998.

[168]	B. Warren, "Gut Health - Ben Warren's top 10 tips for a healthy gut.," 19 Aug 2016. [Online]. Available: https://www.youtube.com/watch?v=SRdEEC4i_3w&feature=youtu.be.
[169]	J. Mercola, The No-Grain Diet, New York, New York: Dutton, 2003.
[170]	Mayo Clinic, "Oral helath: A window to your overall health," 4 June 2019. [Online]. Available: Mayoclinic.org/healthy-lifestyle/adult-health.
[171]	B. D. M. Feldman, "Gateway to Health. Heal your mouth. Heal your body.," 2020. [Online]. Available: Secure.gatewaytohealtyseries.com.
[172]	Gateway to Health, "Gateway to Health," 2020. [Online]. Available: secure.gatewaytohealthseries.com.
[173]	John Hopkins Medicine, "Liver: Anatomy and Functions," [Online]. Available: https://www.hopkinsmedicine.org/health/conditions-and-diseases/liver-anatomy-and-functions. [Accessed 10 May 2021].
[174]	Wikipedia.org, "Appendix (anatomy)," [Online]. Available: https://en.wikipedia.org/wiki/Appendix_(anatomy).
[175]	J. Levy, "Poop: What's Norman, What's NOT + 7 Steps to Helathy Pooping," 19 June 2018. [Online]. Available: draxe.com/health/poop.
[176]	S. Watson, "How long does it take to digest food? All about digestion," 7 October 2019. [Online]. Available: Helathline.com/health/how-long-does-it-take-to -digest-food.
[177]	J. Mercola, "Gut Bacteria a Key to Health," 02 October 2017. [Online]. Available: articles.mercola.com.
[178]	O. Grisham, "Why do Dogs Smell our Crotch," 8 April 2019. [Online]. Available: https://www.animalwised.com/why-do-dogs-smell-our-crotch-1768.html.
[179]	A. Talas, Director, Life on Us: A Microscopic Safari. [Film]. 2014.
[180]	Z. Bush, 2020. [Online].
[181]	S. D. C. Fair, San Diego, CA, 2019.
[182]	D. Main, "Tech & Science," 02 February 2016. [Online]. Available: Tech & Science.
[183]	H. Farrell, R. Jimenez-Flores, B. Bleck, E. Brown, J. Butler, L. Creamer, C. Hicks, C. Hollar, K. Ng-Kwai-Hang and H. Swaisgood, "Nomenclature of the proteins fo cows'milk -- sixth revisioin.," J Dairy Sci, pp. June, 87(6): 1641-74, 2004.
[184]	A. Arnarson, "A1 vs. A2 Milk - Does It Matter?," 14 March 2019. [Online]. Available: Healthline.com/nutritin/a1-vs-a2-milk.
[185]	H. Leese, "What does an embryo need?," Human Fertility (Camb), pp. 180-85. Review., 2003, Nov 6(4).
[186]	E. Suni, "Circadian Rhythm," 20 September 2020. [Online]. Available: https://www.sleepfoundation.org/circadian-rhythm. [Accessed 10 May 2021].
[187]	J. Mercola, "Yes, you can die from a "broken heart" and optimism makes you live longer," 12 Jamuary 2017. [Online].
[188]	P. e. a. Zaninotoo, "Sustained enjoyment of life and mortality at older ages: analysis if the English Longitudinal Study of Ageing," 13 December 2016. [Online].
[189]	M. Hyman, "How to Protect Yourself from COVID-19: Supporting Your Immune System When You May Need it Most," 17 March 2020. [Online]. Available: https://drhyman.com/blog/2020/03/17/protect-yourself-from-covid-19/?utm_source=Broken+Brain+1+%2B+2+%-28Combined+List%29&utm_campaign=27993a7137-EMAIL_CAMPAIGN_2018_03_29_COPY_01&utm_medium=email&utm_term=0_c903b97dee-27993a7137-119565761&mc_cid=27993a7137.
[190]	S. Ekberg, "CoronaVirus (COVID 19) Top 10 Vitamin C Foods you Must Eat," March 2020. [Online]. Available: https://youtu.be/BzpaALfeR2g.
[191]	A. Gibbons, "Evolution of Diet," National Geographic Magazine.

[192]	M. Joel Fuhrman, The End of Heart Disease, The Eat to Live Plan to Prevent and Reverse Heart Disease, New York: HarperCollins Publishers, 2016.
[193]	A. Lamb, Director, *Un-Inflame Me: Reversing the American Diet & Lifestyle.* [Film]. 2017.
[194]	J. K. Black, N.D., The Anti-Imflannation Diet and Recipe Book.
[195]	"Religion and Health Study Progress," *Adventist Health Studies Report 2008: V: 5.,* 2008.
[196]	T. C. Campbell, The China Study.
[197]	N. n. d. USDA, 2015.
[198]	J. Hari, Interviewee, *Chasing The Scream.* [Interview]. 2019.
[199]	J. Lusk and J. Fox, "Consumer Demand for Mandaatory Labeling of Beef from Cattle Administered Growth Hormones or Fed Genetically Modiied Corn.," *Journal of Agriculture and kApplied Economics,* 2002, April.
[200]	R. R. Bollinger, A. S. Barbas, E. L. Bush, S. Lin and W. Parker, "Biofilms in the large bowel suggest an apparent function fo the human vermilform appendix," *Journal of Theoretical biology,* pp. 826-831, 2007.
[201]	D. Mann, *Newsweek,* 2 February 2016.
[202]	*Environmental Sciences Europe.*
[203]	L. A. Tucker, "Caffeine Consumption and Telomere Length in Men and Women of the National Health and Nutrition Examination Survey (NHANES)," *Nutrition and Metabolism,* p. 10, 2017.
[204]	W. W. Li, Eat to Beat Disease, New York, Boston: Grand Central Publishing, 2019.
[205]	J. McClain, D. Hayes, S. Morris and K. Nixon, "Adolescent Binge Alcohol Exposure Alters Hippocampel Progenitor Cell Cell Proliferation in Rats: Effects on Cell Cycle," *Journal of Comparative Neurology 519, No 13,* pp. 2697-2710, 2011.
[206]	"20 facts about obesity," [Online].
[207]	H. Nichols, "Medical Newss Today," 27 December 2016. [Online].
[208]	D. Karl, "A year without food," 24 JUly 2012. [Online]. Available: abc.net.au/science/articles 2012/07/24/3549931.htm.
[209]	J. Mercola, "20 Resolutions for 2020," January 2020. [Online]. Available: media.mercola.com.
[210]	L. Cordain, "Cereal grains: humanity's double-edged sword.," *World Rev Nutr Diet,* pp. 84:19-73, 1999.
[211]	D. Feldman, "Dave Feldman - The Dynamic Influence of a High Fat Diet on Cholesterol Variability," 24 March 2017. [Online]. Available: youtube.com/watch?v=jZu52dulqno.
[212]	J. Mercola, "Mercola Take Control of Your Health," 13 February 2020. [Online]. Available: articles.mercola.com/sites/articles/achive/2020/13/alzheimers-meal-plan.aspx?.
[213]	M. Hyman, "10 Day Reset," [Online]. Available: https://cdn.shopify.com/s/files/1/0020/1008/7522/files/10-day-reset-free.pdf?9174.
[214]	Sasaki, "High blood pressure and the salt intake of the Japanese.," pp. 313-324..
[215]	Rouse, Armstrong and Beilin, "The relationship of blood pressure to diet and lifestyle in two religious populations," pp. 65-71..
[216]	W. H. Organization.
[217]	"Flax nutrition, glycemic index, acidty and serving size," [Online]. Available: https://foodstruct.com/food/seeds-flaxseed.
[218]	A. B. J. M. O. T. H. Keys, The biology of human starvation (2 volumes)., St. Paul, MN.: University of innesota Press, 1950.

[219]	e. a. Rosenbaum, "Long-term persistence of adaptive thermogenesis in subjects who have maintainted a reduced body weight.," *American Journal of Clinical Nutrition. ,* pp. October;88)4): 906-12, 2008.
[220]	E. a. Sims, "Endocrine and metabolic effects of experimental obesity in man.," *Recent Prog Horm Res.,* pp. 29:457-96, 1973.
[221]	F. Benedict, "Human vitality and efficiency under prolonged restricted diet," 1919. [Online]. Available: Https://archive.ort/details/humanvitalityeffoobeneuoft.. [Accessed 25 April 1015].
[222]	M. e. a. Bliwise, "HIstorical change in the report of daytime fatigue," *Sleep,* pp. Jul;19(6):462-4, 1996.
[223]	Wikipedia, "Insulin index," 10 Aug 2020. [Online]. Available: https://en.wikipedia.org/wiki/Insulin_index. [Accessed 30 9 2020].
[224]	"Suet," [Online]. Available: https://en.wikipedia.org/wiki/Suet.
[225]	U.S. Department of Health and Human Sersvices and U.S Department of Agriculture, "Key Rocommendations: Components of Healthy Eating Patterns," Dietary Guidelines for kAmericans, 8th Edition, December, 2015.
[226]	P. Benjamin Bikman, "Insulin Resistance and Obesity Make You Sick, Vulnerable to Infections," 5 12 2020. [Online]. Available: https://youtu.be/L21Pdyjqwto.
[227]	J. Fung and Moore, Jimmy, The Complete Guide to Fasting, Victory Belt Publishing, 2016.
[228]	"New Year's Resolutions Statistics (2021 Updated)," 30 December 2020. [Online]. Available: https://discoverhappyhabits.com/new-years-resolution-statistics/.
[229]	J. LaLannne, "Jack LaLanne THe Godfather of Fitness," 2011. [Online]. Available: https://jacklalanne.com/about/. [Accessed 29 April 2021].
[230]	Healthwise, "Healthy Eating: Overcoming Barriers to Change," 21 Aug 2019. [Online]. Available: Healthy.kaiserpermanente.ort/southern-california/health-wellnes/health-encyclopedia/he.zx-3327#zx3328.
[231]	Sleep Foundation, "What is Circadian Rhythm?," [Online]. Available: https://www.sleepfoundation.org/page/5?s=circadian+rhythm&op=Search.
[232]	C. DerSarkissian, "Fecal Transplant: What You Should KNow," 30 May 2019. [Online]. Available: webmd.com.
[233]	D. N. Campbell-McBride, Interviewee, *A Special Inerview with Dr. Natasha Campbell-McBride.* [Interview].
[234]	Healthwise, "Healthy Eating for Children," 21 Aug 2019. [Online]. Available: healthy.kaiserpermanente.org/southern-california/health-wellness/health-encylopidia/he.tn9188#tn9189.

Index

T

Taubes, Gary 70, 89
teeth 220, 221, 222
Telomeres 143
testosterone 41, 57, 62, 80
The Atkins diet 49
The Cancer Code 162
The Great Cholesterol Myth 60
The Ornish diet 49
The Standard American Diet (SAD) 10
The Zone diet 49
tiredness 207
Too much protein 77
Tooth decay 95
toxins 57, 224, 257, 270
Toxins 175, 181, 256
Traditional diet 49
Trans fats 151, 287
triglycerides 59, 60, 63, 64, 66, 67, 68, 69, 70, 152, 156, 193, 194, 198
Turmeric 288, 290

U

ulcerative colitis 95
Ulcerative colitis 232
ulcers 52, 95, 96
unhealthy food 292
Unsaturated fats 46
U.S. Dietary guidelines 124

V

Varicose veins 52, 96
vegan 11, 56, 74, 75, 161
Vegan 6, 159
vegans 54, 55, 78, 83, 85, 88
Vegetarian 6, 55, 297
vegetarians 53, 54, 55, 78, 88, 138, 241
vitamin C 290
Vitamin C 284
vitamin D 57, 62, 81, 86, 95, 128, 198, 205, 206, 207, 208, 209, 211, 255, 265, 281, 284
Vitamin D 4, 57, 129, 205, 206, 207, 208, 284, 288, 289
vitamin K2 288, 289

Vitamin K2 44, 81, 82, 203, 204, 205, 282
vitamins 224

W

Wahls, Terry 11, 168, 170, 174, 186
Waist- to-hip ratio 33
water 1, 2, 3, 29, 30, 35, 51, 65, 137, 144, 151, 156, 166, 167, 182, 187, 189, 193, 213, 225, 226, 231, 237, 248, 253, 257, 274, 283, 288, 291, 292
weight ix, 2, 7, 14, 15, 16, 17, 18, 19, 20, 21, 22, 24, 25, 28, 33, 37, 38, 39, 43, 48, 49, 51, 60, 74, 76, 77, 87, 88, 90, 91, 97, 98, 99, 104, 106, 123, 133, 134, 135, 136, 140, 143, 152, 181, 192, 193, 194, 229, 251, 254, 255, 269, 282
Weight ix
weight loss 15, 17, 18, 19, 20, 21, 24, 25, 39, 123, 188, 193, 251
wheat 241, 242
Wheat 84, 106, 107, 108, 109, 185, 237
Wheat and Other Grains 106
wheat products 292
William P. Castelli 272
wrinkles 2, 203, 204, 205, 275

Y

yogurt 288, 289
Yogurt 44

Z

zinc 289, 290